*For Ann &
with best
Brian Dorman*

GW00320383

The Tree, The Boat
and the Broken Leg

The story of 'Cherub'

Brian Dorman

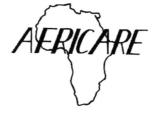

AFRICARE

Published by
Africare
11 Brookeborough Avenue
Carrickfergus
Co Antrim
BT38 7LG
N Ireland
Website: www.besaniya.com

ISBN 0-9553280-0-4
ISBN 978-0-9553280-0-8

CONTENTS

ACKNOWLEDGEMENTS

I want to particularly thank the following for their help with this book.

My wife, Hazel, for the long hours of typing.

Ken McDonald and Laura Collins for proof reading.

Richard Traynor and The Dargan Press for advice
and help in preparing the book for printing.

David Gamble for the cover design.

For I was hungry and you gave me something to eat,

I was thirsty and you gave me something to drink,

I was a stranger and you invited me in.

I needed clothes and you clothed me,

I was sick and you looked after me,

I was in prison and you came to visit me.

Matthew 25:35,36

INTRODUCTION

This book is the story of Cherub – Child Health Education and Rehabilitation Unit, Besaniya – a unit set up in Uganda for the assessment, referral for surgery or other treatment, and rehabilitation of disabled children. It is also the story of what can be achieved by people who had little idea at the time of what they were getting into, but were willing to respond to need.

Cherub doesn't function in isolation, it is part of a broader work. It is based at the Besaniya Children's Home at Mukono. Africare, a small NI based organisation, is the funding agency for Cherub, and also for the Besaniya Children's Programme (which includes the children's home), and ECM (Evangelical Christian Ministries, Uganda), working closely with the national church not only to run missions but to develop effective training programmes for leaders and others. ECM also undertakes pioneering work on some of the more remote islands in Lake Victoria. This is all work that has resulted in blessing. Despite limited resources, the commitment of our workers has enabled us to achieve results beyond anything we could have imagined.

In the Besaniya Children's Home, 34 children are cared for in a Christian family environment. In addition to giving them the security they need, we try to educate and train them effectively, realising their potential and preparing them for the future. As older boys move out, younger children can be admitted. It is here that Cherub has also been developed as we saw the benefit of bringing disabled children, even for a short time, into the Besaniya 'family' and sharing facilities.

I have been responsible for the work of Africare for around 20 years now, with my wife Hazel running the office and dealing with all the administration and finance. What started as part time work soon took over our lives, and we certainly never envisaged being in the position we are now.

'What good is it, my brothers, if a man claims to have faith but has no deeds? Can such faith save him? Suppose a brother or sister is without clothes and daily food. If one of you says to him, "Go, I wish you well; keep warm and well fed", but does nothing about his physical needs, what good is it?' James 2:14-16

The above verses have been an inspiration and motivation to us. I seem to have spent my life doing things I couldn't have imagined or feel ill equipped for. But while it can be a burden it's also a great privilege and it's been thrilling to see so much change take place over the years.

'Jesus replied, "Go back and report to John what you hear and see; The blind receive sight, the lame walk, those who have leprosy are cured, the deaf hear, the dead are raised, and the good news is preached to the poor."'
Matthew 11:4,5

This passage has also been influential in bringing home to us the breadth of Christ's ministry, and in effect giving us a list of 'targets'. When we were first made aware of the needs of disabled children in Uganda, these verses were quoted and clearly showed us once more the need to deal with these physical needs if we were truly to accept that as an example instead of, as has too often been the case, simply bringing words.

In establishing the work of Cherub we've depended on the help of many people. They have provided funds, worked in Uganda, or given support and encouragement in other ways. We are deeply grateful to all of you. Some who helped are mentioned in this story. Others wished to remain anonymous. We are grateful to all of you, and I want this book to serve as a thank you to everyone who gave their time, skills and resources to make it all possible.

1.

AFRICA'S PROBLEMS

For long periods of time, most people give little thought to Africa; then there will be another disaster, natural or man made, and some will respond by helping, some by saying "here we go again", and thinking that our help can't make any difference, and some by making genuine attempts to find solutions. I've lost track of how many different solutions I've heard suggested for Africa's 'problems', and sometimes wonder how much difference they really make. But Africa is a vast continent, with dramatic variations across the different countries in their climate, landscape, natural resources, political structures and many other factors. There isn't a single solution, and I wonder too how different some of their 'problems' are from those experienced by the rest of the world. How much of Africa's suffering is a result of human nature, often compounded by other factors.

In more recent years, there have been a number of high-profile attempts to raise funds and awareness of African issues. This can cause controversy, some people thinking big injections of cash can solve some of the difficulties, others thinking it can make things worse. There are also the ongoing arguments about government help, however well intentioned, serving to prop up corrupt regimes instead of getting through to the people who really need it. I don't claim to have the answer. What I do know is that where there's suffering, people need our help. When their suffering is alleviated, then long term solutions can be sought.

Very recently, while following in the papers another round of debate about the most effective way to help, I read of Africa's problems being blamed on their immorality, indiscipline and lack of work ethic. What a sweeping generalisation! Just look around, how different is this really from the rest of the world, and from the direction our own society seems to be heading. This attitude of generalising takes the well publicised problems of Africa and makes the assumption that it is representative of all that happens there, thus ignoring so much that is positive, the many success stories of modern Africa. Just because it's all so different, don't make the mistake of assuming they can't do anything right or make effective decisions for themselves. It's too easy to use a negative and highly critical view of Africa as an excuse to do nothing – "they've brought it on themselves, so why should I feel responsible." Of course, no Christian can adopt this attitude, can they?

I have experience of working in Africa for very many years, but realise that my knowledge is still very limited. With Africare we have been very fortunate in having the opportunity, and the necessary support, to work with some of the neediest people, free from government or other interference, and have been able to ensure that everything we spend goes directly to those we want to help. This is one of the advantages of being a small agency, fully in control of what we are doing. There is a need for the big agencies too, who can respond to the major problems and disasters, but they face a whole new set of difficulties which we thankfully haven't had to deal with.

We haven't been working in isolation though. It's been a privilege to meet and sometimes co-operate with and work alongside some outstanding people who have made a big impression on everyone they have come in contact with. We're in an era when Africa has become more 'accessible' than ever before. It's easy for us to get on a plane, go out for a few weeks to help with a particular project, and fly home again. I don't want to undervalue the work done by short term volunteers and work teams, we've often needed their help, but in everything we do we have been dependent on the ground work done by those who were willing to commit a large part of their life (or often all of it) to working in difficult and hazardous situations, and staying long enough to develop a fuller understanding and be able to make a real difference. It's because of the pioneering work of many others that we are now able to work there, and I never want to claim that any of the results we are seeing are due to us; often we are only finishing off what someone else started many years before.

We're also in an age when people want instant gratification. When they do something, they want to see results. Of course, some parts of our work are easy to quantify – the number of disabled helped for example, or numbers treated at a clinic. But we follow a long line of people who worked faithfully for years, perhaps never seeing results but never doubting that God had called them to that work. The results may have come long after they were gone. Too few now retain that vision, the willingness to commit themselves and their resources in faith. There must be effective stewardship and accountability, waste must be avoided, but we shouldn't be so eager to judge 'results' by our own criteria. I've been fortunate in getting to know quite a few people who set an example of service which speaks volumes to others. Think of the people they work amongst; they are used to people bringing them words, but sometimes not much else. Imagine what it means when someone is prepared to work alongside them for years on end regardless of personal cost. All kinds of help is needed, some of it easy to provide, some of it difficult, but so much has depended on the personal sacrifice and commitment of a relatively small number who have opened up the opportunities which now exist.

And who were these people who were willing to make such sacrifices? I won't start to name them here, but would urge you to read more of the background to work and mission in Africa; like me, I hope you'll find it an inspiration. But remember that not all of them were from the west; not all were sent to Africa from somewhere else. Consider against those allegations of African's 'immorality, indiscipline and lack of work ethic' those nationals also prepared to put service before selfish considerations. They are the ones we don't hear much about. I am fortunate in having known some of them, of being told the stories of others, and seeing the results of their commitment. Many people around the world are making genuine efforts to help with problems in Africa, but don't lose sight of the fact that many Africans too are striving to help with the sufferings experienced by their neighbours.

Sometimes those with the least understanding of Africa make the most noise about what they think should be done. The more I see of Uganda in particular, the more I realise I still don't understand. What I do know is that having seen some of their suffering, I must respond. Even among Christians, how many of us are truly willing to put the needs of others first? What do we truly aspire to? Is it the relief of others in need, or our own personal ambitions? I can't point the finger, I too have so much more than those I've worked amongst in Uganda, but as a Christian I can't rest easy knowing that they are experiencing difficulty and I have the means to help.

2.

DONALD and UNA BROWNLIE

Although never involved with the work of Besaniya or Cherub, I can't understate their influence on all that has taken place, as it's because of them that Hazel and I visited Uganda in the first place. We had known them in Malawi, but over the years since leaving there hadn't had much contact. That changed when they went to work at Mengo Hospital in Kampala with CMS, and we responded to one of Donald's letters seeking help with putting in a water supply to the hospital. The mail was slow and unreliable, so I thought I would phone Donald to ask if there was anything I could do to help. At the time, I had no idea how unreliable the phone service was, so simply took it for granted when I rang the number and Donald answered. I only found out later that the phone had never worked since being installed in the Brownlie's house, and it came as a complete surprise when it rang!

When we offered to help with Donald's scheme to pump water to the hospital, I had in mind making a donation. I certainly hadn't expected it to lead to us visiting Uganda. Having stayed with the Brownlies and seen the problems faced by the hospital, we determined to do whatever we could to help, and for some years we sourced equipment and drugs, and became regular visitors. Although eventually the focus of our work moved away from Mengo as Besaniya and ECM continued to grow, Donald remained a close friend and major influence. Donald is no longer with us now, and it was only when he became ill that I realised I had never told him just how much he had meant to us. Thankfully, I had the opportunity to tell him, just a few days before he died, how much of an influence he had been on all of our work, and how much had grown out of his having persuaded us to visit Uganda – and also how much his friendship had meant to me personally.

3.

SAMUEL SSEKKADDE

A major influence as we developed our work in Uganda has been Samuel Ssekkadde, now Bishop of Namirembe. In 1984, on our first visit to Uganda, we were staying with the Brownlies at Mengo Hospital – and finding out for ourselves how bad things were in Uganda under Obote. We really had little idea what we were about to encounter when we went to visit the Brownlies.

I was fortunate in being able to borrow an old car which had been 'pensioned' off by CMS. One day, driving down into the centre of Kampala from Mengo, I saw a man in a clerical collar walking by the roadside, and stopped to give him a lift. He introduced himself as Canon Samuel Ssekkadde, principal of the Namugongo Theological College. I had heard about the college, as a short time before there had been a massacre there, but I knew little about the background, or where the college was. However, before we could talk much, we were confronted at a road junction by three apparently very angry gunmen – unfortunately an all too common occurrence at that time. It's hard to know what to do in such situations. There was a policeman directing traffic, and he seemed to distract them. I thus took the opportunity to take off as fast as the old car would go, and thankfully no one started shooting.

I was able to arrange to visit Samuel at Namugongo, and saw for myself some of the aftermath of what had happened there. I heard harrowing accounts of the torture and murder of the previous principal, and how others had suffered. Samuel and his wife Allen were living in quite basic conditions, and Allen was recovering from cancer surgery. We talked at length about the difficulties facing the church in those dark days, and it was through those discussions that ECM has its' origins. We certainly didn't realise then that we would end up working so closely together to deal with the problems we'd

15

identified. On returning home, I sought medical advice and was able to send out drugs to Allen. Thankfully, despite all they've come through, they both remain in good health and are actively involved in many aspects of the work of the Church of Uganda.

Samuel has been able to visit us a number of times in N Ireland, and his wife has also been here. They are very busy people, and we don't see so much of them now but Samuel's commitment to ECM remains undiminished, and it's to Samuel that I would still turn for advice when we face problems.

4.
JOHN and DAISY CROSS

In the early days of our work in Uganda, when I visited the country I usually stayed at Mengo Hospital with the Brownlies. As Besaniya developed, I occasionally stayed there, then, when the Brownlies left Uganda, I would stay at Besaniya and occasionally visit Mengo. It was on one of these brief visits that I met the Crosses.

I'd been in Uganda just a few days when I arrived at Mengo on the back of our Besaniya pick-up truck. As I climbed from the truck in the Mengo car park, I spoke to one of the Mengo workers. I then heard someone, who sounded American, asking "is that an Ulster accent?" When I confirmed that it was, I was asked if I could help them find Brian Dorman! They then introduced themselves as John and Daisy Cross; they were visiting Uganda to look at the possibility of helping with orphans. They also, through their 'Upper Room' charity, helped with the Aids counselling work at Mengo, and had looked at some of the literature we sent out. They were told they should talk to me about orphans, and that I sometimes visited the hospital – at which point I arrived! The surprises didn't stop there. They had left Northern Ireland for Canada in 1948, the year I was born. John had lived just a few streets from my home in Belfast, and attended the same school and church.

I'm always looking for help with our work, so when I heard they had an interest in orphans I wanted to show them Besaniya. However there wasn't time for this as their visit was almost at an end. They did say though that on their way home they were stopping off in Ireland to visit relatives. I then found that they would be staying very close to my own home in Carrickfergus, and would still be there when I got back. We thus had the opportunity to talk at more length about the work.

From this meeting, a number of possibilities opened up. It meant a lot to us that someone so widely travelled, and with so much experience of work in the mission field, was willing to become involved with our projects and give us their support. Since then, they have made a number of visits to Uganda and on occasion I've been able to go with them. They aren't young, but have never lost their enthusiasm or vision, and I've been impressed by their willingness to continue to undertake demanding journeys. They've gone on to become very important to our work, being directly responsible for finding financial support as well as giving us a lot of encouragement. As a direct result of their help, the scope of our work in Uganda is now much broader than would otherwise have been possible – meaning that many more people have been helped. They are keen evangelicals, but also recognised the need to deal with humanitarian problems such as poverty, illness or disability if an effective witness is to be maintained.

5.

PATRICK

ECM had its origins in my first meetings with Samuel Ssekkadde, when we discussed the problems facing the church in Uganda. We started to deal with these problems by undertaking some translation and publishing to address the serious lack of material available in the Luganda language. Training was also a priority, and we began to address this by involving Evangelical Ministries. Through this early work, ECM Uganda was set up under a Ugandan board chaired by Samuel Ssekkadde. The first full time worker was Patrick Wakkonyi, recruited by Samuel. Patrick's job was to co ordinate the work, and it was he who started to develop the network of associates. Patrick's background was as a mechanic/welder, but he was very active in his own church, and had completed various short training courses with other agencies.

Patrick showed remarkable commitment and determination, and when Sam Mutumba also joined ECM they made a very strong team. From the start the emphasis with ECM was on the nurture of converts; we had seen far too many examples of evangelism with neither adequate preparation or follow up. Patrick and his family moved into a house we rented for them, and he put all his energy into building up the work. When Samuel Ssekkadde was appointed bishop of Namirembe and moved into the residence near the cathedral, he gave ECM use of an office which they continue to use.

Although a separate work to Besaniya or Cherub, there are useful links. In particular, ECM now has a widespread network of workers, including those on the islands, who can help locate children who might benefit from treatment in Cherub. Also, just as Sam continues to be involved with management of ECM while working at Besaniya, so we have made use of Patrick's experience and vision as part of the management team overseeing all of our work. We want ECM, Besaniya and Cherub to be different strands of a common work, rather than functioning in isolation. This can bring substantial benefits, including for example, when we send out people with particular skills or gifts and they can be used across the different parts of the work.

ECM developed steadily with literature work, training programmes and missions, but funding was always very tight. We were fully stretched building up Besaniya, still had various medical responsibilities, and found it difficult to build a support base for ECM. We could certainly see the need for it, but hadn't anything to show to potential donors in the way that we had with Besaniya, or with medical work. It was a problem when we would start something, then have to go back and stop it when money ran out. I am thankful that Patrick and Sam continued to work faithfully with ECM despite all the problems, when they could probably have done much better elsewhere; they have been selfless in their service. Sam continued to teach, so wasn't totally dependent on us. Patrick however, while still doing some part time welding for example, was almost totally dependent on what he received from us – and we couldn't pay him very much.

Patrick's determination meant he was constantly pushing us to do more. He didn't like the idea of us paying rent for a house, and encouraged us to consider building a house for ECM. This seemed a good idea, and we started looking around for a suitable plot – eventually buying a piece of land not far from Namirembe. At last we had a 'project' which we could try to get support for, rather than a work which could be difficult to describe to people or have them identify with. Support for ECM only really started to grow when people who had been to Uganda saw for themselves how effective the work was becoming.

Once the land was purchased we had to think about what to build. We drew up preliminary plans for a house, but when Patrick said 'house' what he really had in mind was a training centre which he and his family could also live in. This kind of thing often happened with Patrick – he pushed everything to the limit, but it was always for the sake of the work so was difficult to argue with. He never gave much thought to personal considerations. We drew up plans for what we thought was an adequate house, planned to allow for extension in the future, and instructed Patrick to start work. When I subsequently visited and looked at the foundations, I found out how little relation this actually had to what was on paper. Patrick's interpretation was that any building should fill the available space, to do otherwise would be wasteful! I have also discovered the futility of trying to argue with Patrick, and eventually a much larger house than we'd originally intended was completed. I hesitate to use the term 'finished' – once there was a roof and walls, Patrick wanted to start getting people in for training. The appearance, or anything related to 'comfort' or 'convenience' didn't come far up Patrick's agenda, and it is a battle to do things which we might regard as important but Patrick sees as superfluous.

That house has been in use for quite a few years now, and many training courses have been run. I have been at some of them, and unless I had seen it for myself I wouldn't have believed the house could have accommodated so many people. Many of the associates are in remote rural areas, and there has been great benefit in having them get together for training. It has also often been their only opportunity for fellowship with their co workers; they can be very isolated for much of the time.

We are now starting to further develop the house with a new office, store, and improved accommodation. No doubt this will develop into another struggle with Patrick over how much should be done; he always wants more space, while I would very much like to see the accommodation and facilities brought up to a higher standard. Maybe we will both be able to get what we want. I certainly don't doubt Patrick's ability to get maximum benefit from any additional space.

When ECM was started it didn't take long to recognise the need for transport. It was some time before we were able to do anything about it; the first machine we bought was a small motorcycle – a 'Bajaj' – for Samuel Ssekkadde. This was an Indian built machine based on an obsolete Japanese design. It had the advantage of being quite cheap, and gave good service. I still remember the day Samuel and I went to collect it in Kampala. First, we needed cash – at that time, inflation was such that very large quantities of money were required to buy anything. We went to a Forex bureau in Kampala, wrote a cheque, and filled a number of bags and a small case with cash.

Many people going shopping needed a bigger bag to carry their money than to carry their purchases. Thieves would walk along the street carrying knives to slash the bottom of bags as they walked past – it was impossible to be inconspicuous with money. Fortunately, we got back to the car safely – we were using an old Church of Uganda pick up truck to collect the machine, which couldn't be ridden till registration formalities were completed.

When we reached the importers, we then had to wait while all the money was counted and eventually wheeled out the shiny new Bajaj. We put it on the back of the pick up truck, and only then realised that we didn't have a rope to tie it down. It's hard to remember now what those days were like. There was poverty, and serious shortages of just about everything. This meant that most things were put to some kind of use, so a piece of rope wasn't something that could be kept in a truck in case it was needed, someone would invariably have taken it away for some other purpose. Sometimes things were used for other legitimate purposes, but anything moveable was also likely to be stolen. I hadn't quite got used to the 'system' at that time, and suggested buying some rope. The cheaper Ugandan alternative however, was to have someone sit on the motorbike on the back of the truck, and give them their taxi fare back to Kampala. Simple but effective.

The Bajaj proved very useful, although it was difficult to persuade the rider to wear a helmet. Safety wasn't a high priority for most people, and they seemed to think the value of the helmet might be better used for something else. Safety is still an issue, expediency often dictating that 'short cuts' are taken in the interests of getting the job done – this can apply with travel, use of tools, electricity etc – and we continue to battle with attitudes which we find hard to understand.

Having seen the value of the Bajaj for transporting Samuel Ssekkadde, with consequent benefit to his work, the next step was to buy motorcycles for Patrick and Sam. We eventually bought two 125cc Hondas, one for Patrick, one for Samuel Ssekkadde, and the Bajaj passed on to Sam. When Samuel became bishop, I don't think it was considered appropriate for him to ride a motorbike, so Sam then got the other Honda. Machines can be costly to maintain however, and ECM always seemed to be very short of money.

Sometimes the bikes were in service, sometimes they weren't. I must say though that while Patrick often pushed us to undertake more work or respond to opportunities, he would never complain. Whatever the conditions or difficulties, he just got on with the job.

It is much improved now. We are still often short of money, but only because everything we get is quickly invested in the work, opening up new fields and taking maximum advantage of every opening. The bikes have long ago worn out. With Sam working as field director and based at Besaniya, there is usually a vehicle available – essential because of the range of his responsibilities. Patrick however had no transport. He never complained, and had never asked for anything to help him personally, but it was obvious the problem he had keeping contact with the more distant associates.

By this time a pattern was established. It still amazes me how much work ECM undertook on a very small budget. We rarely had 'surplus' money to enable us to buy something, but if we defined a need, someone would often respond. I decided the time had come to buy a vehicle for Patrick and having made this known, we were very soon given some money. I spoke to Patrick about it, and asked him to look around for a small pick up truck. My aim was that it would be for personal transport; I didn't consider a motorcycle as I could see the benefit of also being able to carry, for example, a generator and projector when he went to visit someone in a remote area.

Patrick was delighted about this, but I should have foreseen what happened next. When Patrick had time to think about it, he came back and tried to convince me that a four wheel drive pick up would enable him to reach more inaccessible areas. I could see the logic to this so agreed. He then tried to convince me that a twin cab pick up would be better, as people or equipment could be carried inside instead of in the open. I conceded that he had a point, and could look for one. At this time, I was still thinking of Patrick's personal transport needs, but he came back again and tried to convince me that if he had a 'minibus' type vehicle instead of a pick up, a team of associates could be carried for missions etc.

I should have realised that from the start Patrick wasn't thinking of his own transport, but of how the work of ECM could benefit. Whatever I might think, anything purchased would be put to virtually constant use in furtherance of the work. This had applied to anything else we had ever bought, from the house to the computer, generators, video etc – nothing was ever idle. I knew the futility of arguing any further with Patrick, so simply told him how much was available and he could buy whatever he thought best. Presumably by this time he already knew what was best, so very quickly came back with a diesel four wheel drive Toyota Hi Ace which he had fitted out with seats – all at what I felt was a very good price. Since then it has proved of enormous value, and has been remarkably durable. It is always fully loaded; the thinking there is that on any journey it would be wasteful to leave any empty space. It has proved an excellent investment and my only concern is that, as with the boat on the lake, ECM is now very dependent on it, and the day will come when it needs to be replaced. I have made a number of journeys with Patrick; it can be a memorable experience. It is never a journey from 'A' to 'B' – there will always be things to deliver or collect, people to see on the way, but it's an education to see the extent of the work he undertakes. Patrick is totally focused on his work as an evangelist and trainer, has enormous energy, and doesn't let himself get diverted. He can be demanding to work with, but is a remarkable and gifted person. He has made a big impression on anyone who has visited Uganda and seen the work of ECM. He is particularly gifted as a leader and carries real authority. It's impressive to see how he can go to, for example, an island on Lake Victoria and take control of a situation, resulting in real change taking place. He's a great motivator who inspires loyalty in those he works with.

He is not the only one in ECM though. He has also been able to choose the right people to take on responsibility in their own areas, and this is making ECM a very strong organisation. And of course everyone has their strengths and weaknesses, and I have always believed that ECM is at its best when Patrick and Sam are able to work together. For a time, the demands of Sam's work with Besaniya and Cherub made it difficult for him to devote much time to ECM, but thankfully that is changing. They are two very different people, but complement each other very effectively, forming a very strong team. Looking at all that has taken place with ECM, it is hard to imagine how anyone else could have done it. And of course Samuel Ssekkadde, from whose original vision it all developed, remains closely involved.

6.
WOBLENZI

The Uganda we work in now is very different to what we encountered when we made our first visit in 1984. Now, there is rapid economic growth, new buildings springing up all over Kampala, and we enjoy a stability that has made it possible for the work to steadily develop. That is only part of the picture though. The visitor to Uganda sees Kampala, with its booming economy, new hotels and shopping centres. What they don't immediately see is that the wealth created is in the hands of a very small number of people.

As they get further from the city a different picture emerges of people in the villages struggling to feed themselves and their families, particularly where family land has been sold to raise money for drugs for Aids sufferers. They see large areas where people's lives have been largely untouched by the prosperity elsewhere in the country. They see people in the villages whose children, instead of being content to live as subsistence farmers or to try to develop the land and make it more productive, are drawn to the bright lights of Kampala. For some, that can lead to success, for most it leads to poverty, misery, crime, Aids.

Then worst of all, they see the terrible suffering in the north with the continuing atrocities of the LRA. A massive humanitarian disaster unfolding just a few hundred miles from Kampala and yet seemingly a world away. Why does this continue in the face of the resources of the Ugandan army? Why isn't the rest of the world doing something about it? Where are the United Nations forces? It is a terrible indictment on a developing country, and on the rest of the developed world, that this can continue.

When we first went to Uganda in 1984, I travelled out with my family – Hazel, Philip and Alan – in response to a request from Donald Brownlie at Mengo Hospital. We had helped send out water pumps, and now Donald wanted me to see the project for myself and perhaps give some help. We knew very little about the situation in Uganda at that time but as the day of our departure drew nearer we kept hearing more warnings. To some extent Uganda had slipped out of the news with the overthrow of Idi Amin. What we didn't realise was that in some ways things had got a lot worse. Some experts warned us against travelling, but we believed it was right to go ahead. There were various obstacles in our path, but we got there and were soon to be shocked by what we saw.

The journey to Uganda was the first time we had encountered Africare. It was a small N Ireland based charity helping support the work being done by Africa Foundation at Moniko Farm, where a number of orphans were cared for. While in Uganda we were able to visit Moniko, and several of the work team members came and stayed with us at Mengo. By that time the weaknesses were appearing in the organisation of Africa Foundation which would eventually lead to Africare breaking the link with them. That's when I joined them, and the development of Besaniya started.

When we arrived in Uganda, first impressions were very bad. The airport was in very poor repair, no lights, bullet holes everywhere, surly and unco-operative officials. It didn't get much better. Signs of war everywhere. There was still evidence of Kampala having at one time been a beautiful city, but now there was devastation. Ruined buildings everywhere, naked beggars and animals searching for scraps in the rubbish piled in the streets. And constant army roadblocks; other than delays they didn't cause us too many problems, but for Ugandans they could make life miserable – stealing from them, wanting bribes to let them through.

At Mengo, we saw a hospital struggling to provide a service to people who mostly couldn't afford to pay. There was a lot for us to take in, it was all so different from anything we'd seen before. We had been unaware of how bad the security situation had become, but that soon changed. We were safe in the hospital compound, but Mengo was on a hill so we could hear what went on all around. The first night, our children wanted to sleep outside in a tent with the Brownlie children. We didn't object, but soon changed our mind when darkness fell and the gunfire started. I've no idea how close it was, but camping soon seemed a very bad idea.

Each night we would hear gunfire, sometimes screams, then in the morning staff would come into the hospital with stories of what was happening in their own areas, and we also saw victims coming in for treatment. Obote's soldiers would move into a selected area, and go from house to house looting whatever they could. If they weren't given enough, they shot the occupier. By day there was an illusion of normality with people going about their business – even in the worst of times, people found ways to survive, and a lot of trade was still taking place. By night, Kampala became a ghost town. Not a light, not a person to be seen. No one dared venture out. No one that is apart from Donald Brownlie, who sometimes persuaded me to come with him.

By this time the water pumps were operating and Mengo already depended a lot on them. There were also frequent power cuts, often due to the very poor state of the local power lines. Donald took it very personally if the pumps stopped working for any reason. They ran all night, filling up a big tank at the hospital ready for work to start in the morning. The spring was some distance from the hospital, and someone slept in the heavily fortified pump house, ready to alert Donald if there was any problem. It wasn't long before something went wrong. The power went off. Instead of waiting till morning, Donald and I went out to investigate. We went to the home of a Uganda Electricity Board worker and Donald somehow persuaded him to come with us. There's no way he would ever have come out at night for anyone else! The end result was the engineer up a pole, working by the light of the car's headlights to restore the power and get the pumps working again.

On another occasion, when we all went to Lake Nabugabu for a short break, Donald and I travelled back to a wedding at Makarere University. We then had to travel out to Nabugabu after dark – not a wise thing to do. By this time many of the soldiers on the road blocks were drunk, so it could be a tense experience.

One event from that period left a particular impression. One night, within the hospital, I saw a woman walking towards the gates carrying the body of her child. We couldn't let her walk back into Kampala alone in these circumstances, so Donald and I got her into the car and drove to her home in the slums. It was a strange experience, the city in darkness and apparently completely deserted. We drove as far into the slums as we could, and then had to walk. I carried the body as the woman led the way. I am sure there were a lot of people around but we couldn't see them and there was no sound. When we reached her house I carried the body inside, laid it down and we came out – I don't think a word was spoken. Everyone at that time lived in fear, not knowing what each night would bring. A number of times I heard people say that even under Idi Amin they were safe at night – but not any more. There was real terror.

One of the first people I met at Mengo was Christopher Wamala, who at that time looked after the pumps. On the day after we arrived, Christopher came to the Brownlie's house to tell us he had just heard his father had been murdered. He wanted to travel home immediately, but came from the notorious Luweero Triangle and Donald said it would be too dangerous for him to travel there alone. At that time foreigners weren't particularly at risk so Donald thought it would be safe for us to take him there. I was very quickly getting to see more of Uganda than I'd bargained for.

We set off out to Woblenzi. This had been a major trading centre, but was now devastated. Few buildings were left undamaged, and most of the inhabitants had fled. We then had to turn on to a minor road to Christopher's village. Because no one dared travel in the area, the road was completely overgrown – in places, the grass was higher than the car and I had to drive with Donald walking ahead to guide me. We kept passing deserted houses; the few people left fled into the bush when they heard a vehicle, fearing it would be soldiers. When we reached Christopher's home, his family had fled too and he had to walk into the bush calling their names. They told us a harrowing story, all too typical for the area, of how the soldiers came to rob them and when they couldn't give them money, Christopher's father was tortured and murdered in front of the family.

I was later to see further evidence of torture. On my next visit to Uganda, when Obote had been overthrown, we were able to travel more freely. I had previously met Misaeri Kauma, bishop of Namirembe, and he asked me to come with him to a confirmation service near Lutete. There were some things he wanted to show me, so on the way to Lutete we stopped at a village where he had known the people. The only person we saw there was a small boy looking through piles of bones hoping to find the remains of his parents. For some years human remains were left in the open. Some said this was because they didn't want to bury people who hadn't been identified. Another reason was that many Ugandans felt that the rest of the world didn't know or care what had happened under Obote, and they wanted them to see the evidence. On other occasions, going to clinics with Donald, we walked along paths lined with bones and often saw skeletons with wires attached, evidence of the methods used to torture them.

Health services were in total disarray, and Donald was trying to re-establish clinics. We helped where we could with drugs and equipment, and saw considerable change over the next few years. My overriding impression at that time was of the sheer scale of the suffering, of how these people had been largely forgotten, and of how inadequate the response was. Thankfully a lot has now changed, and yet I see a parallel with the problems in the north, people suffering on a scale we find hard to imagine.

It was against this background that Besaniya was started. Simeon Weihler, who had worked for Africa Foundation, was effectively 'adopted' by Africare, when we backed his plans to build Besaniya. Only a small number of children could be cared for, particularly in the early years, but the alternative was to do nothing. We as supporters of the work could have little understanding of the enormous difficulties faced by Simeon in getting it all started. Like a number of others, his commitment and determination were such that he remained there through the worst of the fighting, and it's on the foundation he laid that all the present work takes place.

7.
THE BARN

The origins of Cherub can be traced back to 1996, in a barn outside Omagh. For years we sent container loads of supplies and equipment to Uganda. Starting with basic 'relief' supplies, we came to concentrate much more on medical equipment, and regularly lifted loads from various hospitals. This we then prepared for shipment in our store in Carrickfergus. We were asked to collect a load near Omagh, but knew little about it other than it being orthopaedic equipment, and that it would need a large lorry. We were fortunate in having free use of a very large furniture lorry, so went off to Omagh to collect it all. This was no easy task – orthopaedic equipment is very heavy and we were limited in the volunteers we could get at short notice. Suffice to say that the small number of us who had to load it all weren't a particularly 'able bodied' bunch and it was a very demanding days work. The quantity of it all certainly took us by surprise, and the lorry was loaded to the roof. Unfortunately, being a furniture lorry it wasn't meant to have such heavy items loaded to such a height and we found that stability was a serious concern. This came to light at a bend over a bridge, but fortunately it didn't overturn and the rest of the journey back to Carrickfergus went smoothly.

When all the boxes were unloaded and set out in rows on the floor, we could see the scale of what had to be done. There were over 45,000 items across a full range of orthopaedic equipment, all needing to be sorted and made up into sets. Usually when we collected equipment from hospitals, much of it would be unsuitable for some reason – unusual sizes, not matching other items, worn out, damaged, incomplete etc. However, in this case not only was everything new, but it mostly made complete sets, covering the full range of sizes where applicable.

It did however, need a lot of work to list it all and prepare it. We got the necessary help and started the task. It was tedious work, and often very cold and uncomfortable. It ended up taking over a year to deal with it all. We then had to decide what to do with it, and after talking to a number of surgeons the bulk of it was made up into three shipments – one for hospitals in Nepal which we sometimes helped with air freight consignments, one for Kiwoko hospital in Uganda, and one for Mengo hospital in Kampala. It was pleasing to hear from Nepal, and from Kiwoko, how useful the equipment was and how quickly it was put to use. With Mengo, while we knew they did orthopaedic work we weren't sure how much of it would eventually be used. However, around this time a new work was developing under CBM at Mengo with a Canadian surgeon, Norgrove Penney, overseeing the Uganda Orthopaedic Project, dealing with disabled children. Norgrove was able to use a lot of what was sent, making up extra instrument sets and using many of the consumables such as plates, screws and implants.

When I next went to Uganda, I was able to visit Mengo and see for myself what Norgrove was doing – and very impressive it was. Not only were many disabled children being helped, but the orthopaedic theatres were being run to a very high standard and providing quality training to Ugandan surgeons. Norgrove would run 'workshops' in which other surgeons gained experience. A 'trainee' surgeon would start by observing, then assist, then carry out the surgery themselves. Norgrove told me of one such workshop when 60 club foot operations were completed in one week – with Norgrove, having got things started, spending much of the time drinking tea and keeping an eye on proceedings.

Norgrove's aim at first had been to treat children in their own areas, using local hospitals. In practice this proved difficult; there were problems with allocation of theatre time, availability of the necessary equipment and skilled help etc, so instead Norgrove developed a 'dedicated' theatre at Mengo. There's a lot of history there too, as the building used was Sir Albert Cook's original operating theatre, dating back to 1897. Over the years, after serving for a long time as the hospital's main operating theatre, it was also used as a library, and it was wonderful to see such a historic building once again serving its original purpose – and also to see it function to such a high standard. The building housing the theatre, and the original hospital wards, is among the oldest buildings still standing in Uganda, and much of the rest of the building has also now been renovated. Norgrove was able to convert the rooms above the theatre into an office and classroom, and equip a small second theatre and preparation area.

In Africa, some things have to be done to a lesser standard than might otherwise be desirable because of the constraints of finance, skills or facilities. However, with orthopaedic surgery there is really only one way to do it, and it's wonderful to see such a high standard applying with the building, equipment and staff. It is setting an excellent example, and also achieving a very high success rate –and very low rate of infection – often with extremely sick children. In fact, Norgrove's personal determination has led to him dealing with a number of 'lost causes' – children who by conventional wisdom should have been beyond help. It has also been impressive to see the complexity of the surgery being undertaken by a number of Ugandan surgeons; what was started at Mengo thus had the opportunity to become much more far reaching.

Seeing what was done at Mengo made a deep impression, and so were sown the seeds which would eventually lead to the starting of 'Cherub'.

8.

SALAAMA

Our interest in disability extends beyond Cherub. Since Besaniya was started we have always wanted to seek out those who were most in need in the hope that we could provide some help. We are particularly interested in projects where we can already see someone making an effort – it's easier to help when there is already some degree of organisation. One day at Besaniya I was told someone wanted to see me. This was nothing new, word gets around when I'm there, and people often turn up looking for help. Most of the time the requests can be ill considered, ill conceived, unrealistic or downright fraudulent. Or, much as we might like to, we are simply unable to help. Occasionally though we may be able to help someone, and Salaama proved to be a fruitful example of co operation.

I got the message and went up to the Besaniya office to meet with a man called Francis. He was blind, and had a particular burden for blind children. He told me about his work at Salaama, where he ran a hostel for blind children. In theory, children placed there should have had fees paid by their parents; in practice, children were often effectively abandoned there – not only were fees not paid, sometimes no one ever came back for them. I didn't think too much at the time about Francis' story. I was used to hearing requests from people who said they wanted to help others but hadn't the capability to back up their ideas. However, Francis left a detailed report and when I got round to reading it I could see how thorough he had been. I think we sent him a modest gift to give him some encouragement – we usually had enough to do finding support for our existing responsibilities. Some time later we were able to visit Salaama. It wasn't very far away but the road was bad so it wasn't very accessible. The hostel was a former school for blind children which had steadily deteriorated since losing its funding. The whole place was now in very poor repair, and the hostel had only six resident children who had to walk to a nearby school.

When we looked around, we could see they were doing their best to keep it all going with inadequate resources, and it was very difficult for them to deal with any repairs or maintenance. We saw a number of things which could be improved very easily, so gave what help we could – including having Besaniya children go there to help with digging and planting. We also started to upgrade parts of the buildings. This process continued, and further help came from donors and work teams. New latrines were provided, roofs repaired, electricity installed, and a playground built. They were able to take in more children; The Upper Room, at the request of the local pastor, helped with the school and soon the whole place had been transformed. The children's spiritual needs were also addressed, with our workers regularly staying there. Now the enrolment is 58 children and the school receives a government grant. This is the kind of project we like to assist with, as we are able to bring them to a point where they are no longer dependent on us.

9.
LEGO

We've been very glad of the help we've received from the many visitors to Besaniya over the years – but not everyone sees it in the same way, and their perception of the work may be different from ours. Visitors have commented on the quality of the food or the state of the children's clothes. Often what they really mean is that the food isn't what they're used to, and it takes time to adjust. The children in Besaniya are very well fed, bearing in mind that we're feeding a large number and are conscious of the cost. Clothing isn't a big concern for us either. We want them to be properly dressed for school, but it's a hot country so warm clothing isn't important, and what may look like rags to visitors may be entirely appropriate for Besaniya. The way the children work and play, any clothes will very quickly be reduced to rags anyway.

Some people still want to donate clothing, but this is unrealistic. In the early days of our work, we did send out large quantities of clothing, but import duty is now very high and anything we require is easily and cheaply available in Uganda. We feel that every child in our care is provided with all they need, however it may look to others. We've seen what happened in the past if a well intentioned visitor gave a new shirt, for example, to one of the boys. If he already has whatever he needs, he'll probably go straight to town and sell the new shirt. I also remember seeing one of the older boys washing Alan Clegg's Toyota. He was wearing a very smart new shirt. He didn't have a sponge to wash the car, so took off his shirt and used that.

People are often surprised at how, even in the midst of poverty, Ugandans can still manage to look smart. During the week, you'll see them wearing what may look like rags but are in fact perfectly adequate. Then, come

Sunday when they're going to church you will see a transformation. The clothes may be old and worn, but they can still take a lot of care with their appearance. We want the Besaniya children to value whatever they have. They are all responsible for washing their own clothes – this is normally done in the mornings before they go to school. An inspection is sometimes required though, as we have found boys taking short cuts in the past and it wasn't unknown for unwashed clothes to be hung out on the lines, to give the appearance that they had been washed.

We have to provide for all the children's needs – we accommodate them, educate them, as well as clothing and feeding them. We also expect them to work, in an attempt to avoid them starting to think everything will come easily. They won't properly value anything we give them which is beyond their needs, and it isn't helpful in encouraging them to become independent. When children come to Besaniya their biggest need is security. Anything else is 'superficial' and of no great importance.

At times we have had a particular difficulty with attitudes to toys. Visitors have often commented on how the Besaniya or Cherub children don't have toys. The reason for this is that we don't think they need them. When a child comes into Besaniya or to Cherub, they become part of a family. It's a strong unit, and the children quickly come to identify with it and form a real bond which transcends tribal or other differences. There is a lot of emphasis on work and on education, but recreation is very important too. Many of the children who come, whether long or short term, haven't been 'socialised', and it's a joy to see them start to relate to other children. They quickly learn to play together, and you will rarely see a child on their own or trying to think of something to do. There are organised games, or various impromptu activities. At times there seem to be no limits to the children's imaginations. Giving toys to individuals would end up stifling their imaginations, or altering their expectations. We try to ensure that everything provided for them at Besaniya encourages them to work together – board games, equipment for table tennis or other sports. The exception can be the library, where some of them tend to go later in the day. There, they can engage in 'quiet' activities – reading, jigsaw puzzles, perhaps chess or draughts. We don't want to do anything to compromise this ability to do things together. I sometimes have to intercept toys sent by visitors who haven't listened to our advice. The one exception is Lego, which has proved a useful educational tool. We always keep a quantity of it there, and it's been a big help in developing the children's skills. We have seen the satisfaction a child derives when they manage to put wheels on something and can push it across the floor. It can also be used in a more structured environment to demonstrate mechanical principles.

I still remember the night Lomokol was brought to Besaniya. He was from Karamoja, an orphan brought to us by a pastor. He was undernourished, with bad open sores. He was also frightened, had probably never seen white faces, and spoke a different language so couldn't communicate with anyone. He slept in my room that night – he'd been brought in quite late. Next day, the older boys dressed his sores, but we then weren't sure what to do with him. Then, to our amazement, one of the younger boys appeared with a box of Lego components and showed them to Lomokol. In a very short time they were both on the floor totally engrossed in putting the bricks together and oblivious to everything else.

Even for sports or other communal activities we've to be careful how much equipment we provide, as they are used to making things for themselves. They can produce very effective footballs using the liners from milk cartons. All kinds of scrap – empty boxes, pieces of electrical cable, bottle tops – can be put to use. It doesn't get any easier though. As Uganda's economy improves, everyone's aspirations change as they see the range of imported goods appearing in the shops. It is difficult for us to teach values when as well as increasing prosperity they see greed all around them. The time is approaching when we need to carefully consider our whole philosophy and strategy for how we care for children. In many ways it is easier with the Cherub children. They are disabled, what they want above anything else is to be like other children. They can then go back to their parents and communities and we don't have the problem of dealing with their changing expectations as they grow older and see more.

From the skills learnt through sports and activities, it's a short step to looking at more practical skills, and for this the Besaniya workshop, farm and forest can be valuable. These children have to make their way in life, and in addition to their formal education, which can at times be rather narrow, we want them to have broader capabilities. At the farm, Myambala, the manager, can give useful instruction. At the forest, they are sometimes put to work clearing the ground, digging, planting – apart from anything else this can burn off excess energy. Then at the workshop, they can be taught how to make things for themselves. It's difficult fitting it all in as we need people with the ability to teach the skills, as well as equipment and materials, but at times the children work on 'projects', each for example producing a small table for themselves. As well as learning skills, they have the satisfaction of having made something for themselves.

We do though see problems in the future encouraging the children to value something which they have made or done for themselves in comparison to something which can be bought – especially when, whatever they might want, there are very tight constraints on what they can realistically hope to be able to pay for in the future.

10.

ALAN WHO?

It came as a shock to us when John Moffett warned us that he was planning to leave Besaniya. It shouldn't have, because he gave us plenty of warning. Also, although John had agreed to go out to Uganda to run Besaniya for a year, he ended up staying for five. We were very grateful to John for this commitment, and the stability he brought to the work by staying for so long. The problem was that because he stayed so much longer than he had originally agreed to, we hadn't given any thought to his eventual replacement.

It was difficult to define the type of person we needed for Besaniya, or to draw up a job description. By now Fred and Mirica Kisitu had been house parents for a number of years and their job was to deal with day to day running of the home and supervision of the children. However, we weren't yet ready to hand over entirely to local control, so still needed someone there as our link who could handle all the finance, deal with repairs and maintenance or any new development work, and provide us with the level of reporting and accountability required. That's what should be involved, but in reality the expectation there was that anyone we sent out would be in overall control, having to take responsibility for just about everything.

We could have tried to draw up a detailed job description, and then tried to find someone to fit it. In reality, it was a case of 'who can we think of.' We needed someone mature and experienced. We weren't so concerned about a person's skills as their ability to understand the work, to fit in, and to cope with all the different relationships. As so often happened we didn't have many options, and there was only one person I could think of who might be suitable. Correction, there were probably quite a few suitable people around, but how many of them would be willing to leave everything behind and go to work at Besaniya?

There are times when I wonder why Alan Clegg was still willing to have anything to do with us. We first met him in 1989, when Hazel, myself, and our boys Philip and Alan went to Mengo Hospital. We had gone to stay with the Brownlies, but space was limited in their house, so Mengo decided we should have a house to ourselves. This was a problem, as there was a lot of pressure on accommodation for hospital staff. Alan, a farmer from Port Laoise in Ireland, had gone out to Mengo with CMS to serve for a couple of years as farm manager for the hospital, which had several hundred acres of land near Mityana. Alan was single, and had been allocated a house of his own within Mengo. When they heard we were coming Alan was asked to move in with the Brownlies so that we could have his house for the two months we would be there. Despite this, we got on well and I was able to visit the Mengo farm with Alan to see what he was doing.

Alan would describe himself as a 'quiet' Christian, he doesn't see himself as a preacher or teacher but tries to set a Christian example in all he does. On this and a subsequent visit it was evident how much Alan cared about the farm workers and others he came in contact with and how much he was prepared to do to try to help them.

I felt we hadn't got off to a very good start by having Alan moved out of his house, but things were to get much worse. The situation in Uganda was still very tense and there was a strong military presence, with several army installations close to Mengo. While out walking, I tried to take a photograph of a building which had originally been modelled on Stormont, in N Ireland. A number of soldiers quickly appeared, and Alan and I were arrested for spying. We were taken away for questioning, and the building we were held in (formerly military intelligence headquarters) still had a lot of blood on the walls giving some idea of what had gone on there. Some of the officers were little more than children, and were heavily armed. Our interrogators seemed convinced that I was a soldier. Unfortunately for Alan, when they heard his accent he was accused of being in the IRA. Although we were later released and able to return to Mengo they had taken whatever we had with us including our cameras, and also held our passports. We had to keep going back each day, and although we involved the British High Commission, in some ways this made things worse. It seemed this was all being done to get us to part with money, and on one occasion a very indirect approach was made suggesting quite a large sum which we couldn't have afforded even if we had been willing. We were determined though not to hand anything over in case that left us open to charges of bribery.

After a worrying four or five days, several very young soldiers arrived at Mengo one evening and gave us back our passports with no further explanation. We never saw our cameras again and weren't too inclined to go looking for them. After all this, it wouldn't have been surprising if Alan would happily have forgotten about us when we left for home.

When Alan completed his time in Uganda and came home to Port Laoise, we had very little contact. We spoke only occasionally. When in Uganda he had been able to visit Besaniya and we could see how much he cared about children. He had visited other projects too, and been deeply touched by some of the work he saw done with disabled children. I think at the time Alan would have seriously considered a request to work at Besaniya, but it didn't arise as we didn't need anyone else there.

Several years passed, with Alan settled into life in Port Laoise. Much of the farm was let out, and Alan was looking around for something to occupy himself, so he started working on picture frames and eventually equipped a workshop. Then one day he got a phone call from me asking if he'd go to Besaniya.

When John Moffett told us he was leaving, Alan's was the only name I could think of. I knew of his previous interest in Besaniya, his concern for children, and his experience of Uganda. I had no idea if he would still be remotely interested. Alan had started working on picture frames in one of the outbuildings at his home, but on the day I phoned him to ask about work in Uganda he had just signed the lease for a shop in a nearby town. He also really didn't think he was competent for the work we wanted him to do – it was so different from anything he had experienced. For anyone else this would have been enough for them to refuse the offer, but not for Alan. Despite all the apparent barriers Alan was in fact willing to go, and almost immediately gave notice on the lease he had just taken out. How many people would have responded in this way? Plans of their own, and asked to do a job they didn't feel capable of, but because he was needed he was willing to do it. Once more, Alan's actions said a great deal more than most Christians say with words.

We had house parents at Besaniya already, and Alan certainly didn't want to take direct responsibility for a home full of children. Also, job titles there can mean a great deal so we had to think carefully. Titles like 'manager' or 'director', whatever our intentions, would have created the perception of him being totally in charge whereas we really wanted him as our representative, letting others get on with their own jobs. We settled on 'projects director', as some development was still taking place and Alan very much wanted a 'hands on' role. Sometimes specialists aren't much use in Africa, what is needed is an all rounder who can tackle a range of tasks. We have always found that a farming background can be a very useful grounding, as they have had to deal with so many different things. As well as any development which might be planned, there was all the repair and maintenance work around Besaniya, and we were also happy for Alan to keep up his links with Mengo and the various CMS personnel he'd come to know while in Uganda before. As long as he was able to represent us when needed, we were happy for him to help others too.

When people were informed that we wanted to send Alan to replace John Moffett, the reaction wasn't always positive. With some justification, they pointed to his apparent lack of relevant experience. My argument was that John Moffett had no relevant experience when we sent him out, it was the usual situation for us of John being the only person available and he went on to do an outstanding job for much longer than we could have hoped. So it was with Alan; if someone suitable with lots of experience with children, or management of a home for example, had offered to go, we'd have sent them – but there wasn't anyone else. What we had was someone with experience of Uganda who was willing to go, and that was enough for me.

There followed a very disruptive period for Alan. He had to wind up the picture framing business and deal with matters relating to the farm and the sale of some land, and prepare to go out to Uganda to do a job which he knew would place great demands on him. I well remember going to Port

Laoise to help him pack away his personal effects, and was there when he turned the key to lock his house and walked away from it. And he wasn't looking back, he was looking forward. He wasn't thinking of what he had given up, of what he was leaving behind, nor did he have any unrealistic ambitions or expectations of what he would achieve in Uganda. He simply wanted to go there and do the job we'd asked him to do.

Alan writes:

"A Sad Story: when we started the Cherub building programme, a man approached me for work as a labourer. I was warned to be careful as he could be light fingered, but decided to give him a chance. He proved to be a good worker, but we soon found he was up to his old ways as tools started to disappear, and we couldn't keep him on.

"I hadn't seen him for five or six months when he arrived at my door one morning to tell me his little boy had died of malaria and that he had no money to bury him. He told me that his son had died because he had no money to buy drugs to treat him. He had no money because he hadn't worked from the time we let him go; he was dismissed because he was dishonest. The little boy had died because his father was a thief.

"I gave him more money to bury the child than it would have cost to buy the drugs to save his life. A sad story, but all too common. Part of the deal for the money was that he would return the property he had stolen, he even got down on his knees to ask for forgiveness, but we have never seen him again."

July 2002:

"I want you to picture in your mind a small boy of about five years wearing a Lizaroff frame (a device for straightening a crooked bone) on his left leg, with a crutch under his arm, playing badminton with no trousers on. That is what Besaniya has come to these days! His name is Musisi and he has been wearing the frame now for more than six months. The bone is now straight, but it has taken longer for it to strengthen sufficiently for him to use his leg normally. His condition was caused by an insect bite which affected the growth plates in his leg, thus causing it to grow abnormally. This is just one of the many different and unusual cases which have been coming through Cherub since it was started just over one year ago.

"As I prepare to leave Besaniya I have mixed feelings. I am sad that I am saying goodbye to a very important and enjoyable chapter in my life. But even apart from getting married and moving on to a new part of my life I feel it is time for me to leave.

"Besaniya has been very good for me. It has given me the chance to put all the experiences of my life into use in a practical way. No university degree could have prepared me for the work that I have had to do here. It has been a hands on, heart on experience; if the heart wasn't in it then the hands couldn't do it.

"My job as projects director has taken me to almost every street and corner in Kampala on more than one occasion. I know most of the shops in Nakasero market, plus most of the market boys who after three years still try to con me every time I go in. I have so much experience of driving in Kampala that I hope I can re-learn good driving practice when I leave, and don't do too much damage in the process."

Some time after leaving:

"I am a quiet Christian. If what I do is a good example to someone else then I reckon that is what God wanted of me. I will always be grateful for the way he used me to establish the caring project in Uganda now known as Cherub.

"When I was asked to return to Uganda, my job as projects director was to build water tanks and other improvements such as storm drains etc. At that time there was absolutely no mention of building a rehabilitation unit for physically disabled kids, yet within five months the project was well under way.

"My initial introduction to disabled kids was way back in 1990 when I visited a project in Mbarara.. Surgery was carried out by visiting surgeons a few times a year and then the kids were given whatever support was available in the area. I remember being humbled and deeply touched by one old man who had carried his grandchild on his back for many days so as to get him some help. I also remember seeing kids who had previously been sitting in the mud because of contracted limbs from polio and other ailments, and now they were able to walk. How wonderful this was and what a major difference it made to the lives of those kids and their families."

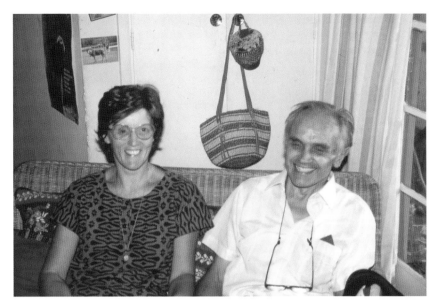

Donald and Una Brownlie

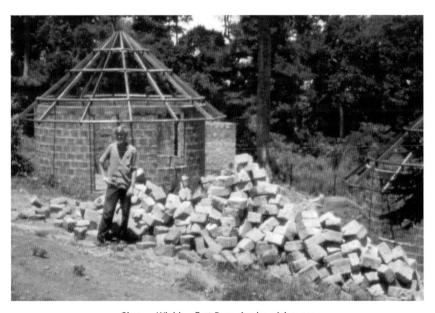

Simeon Wiehler, first Besaniya boys' houses

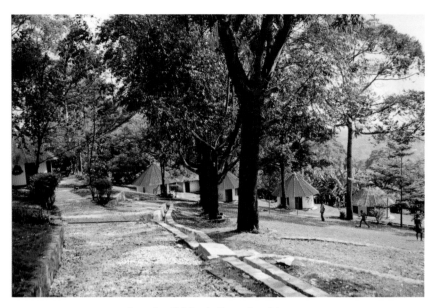

Besaniya Children's Home, boys' houses

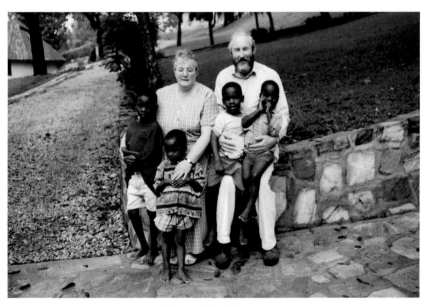

Brian and Hazel Dorman

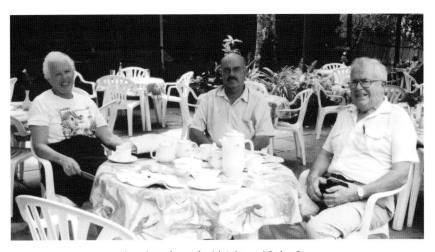

Alan Clegg (centre) with John and Daisy Cross

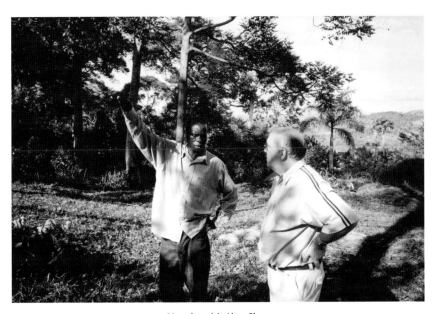

Musoke with Alan Clegg

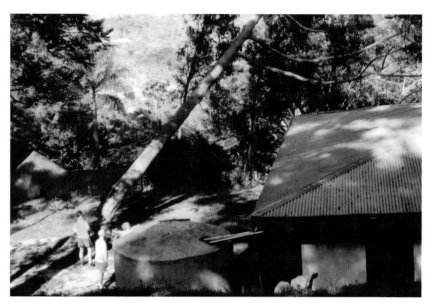

Felling the tree at the Cherub site

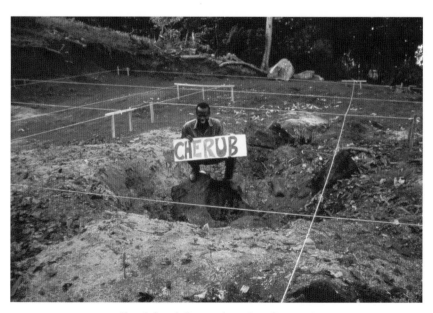

Cherub foundations and remains of tree root

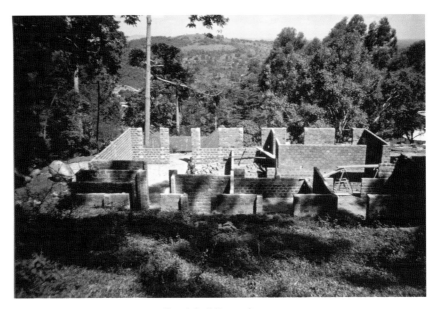

Cherub building under way

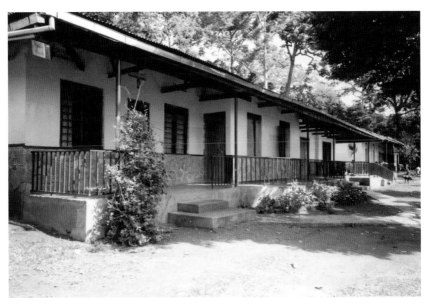

Besaniya main building with Cherub beyond

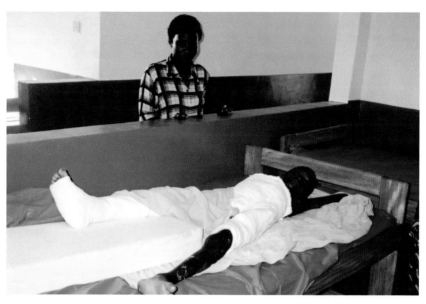

James, the first Cherub patient

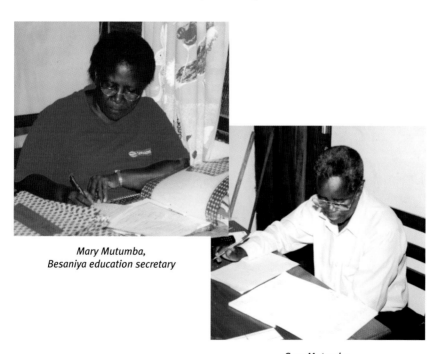

*Mary Mutumba,
Besaniya education secretary*

*Sam Mutumba,
Africare field director*

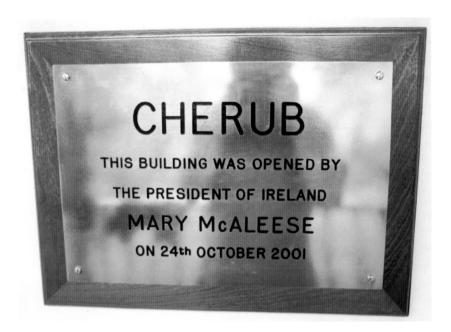

CHERUB

THIS BUILDING WAS OPENED BY

THE PRESIDENT OF IRELAND

MARY McALEESE

ON 24th OCTOBER 2001

Cherub Opening

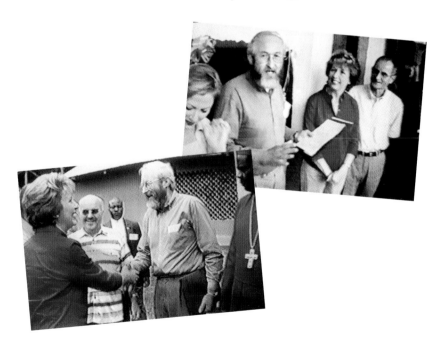

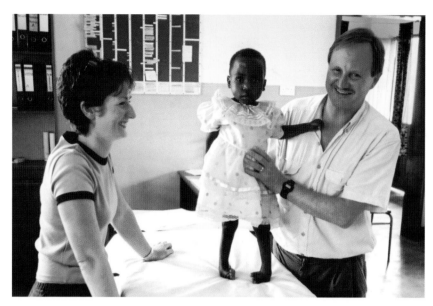

Florence Mawhinney and Norgrove Penny

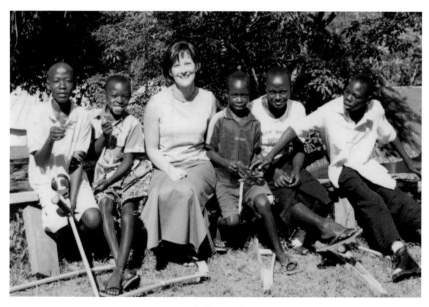

Danielle Mondor

11.

THE IDEA

I had a particularly enjoyable trip to Uganda in March 2000, travelling out with John and Daisy Cross. Instead of having to deal with problems or walking into a crisis, we spent a lot of time looking around with Alan Clegg at how well everything was doing. This however caused us to question what we should do next. The easiest way forward would have been to leave things as they were. Besaniya was 'complete', it had been built to what seemed to be the optimum size, with any extra resources being used for external sponsorship. It all seemed to be running smoothly, and all we had to do was transfer out the budget each month and let them get on with it. We didn't even have to worry too much about finance, as the support from donors matched what was being spent. How thankful I am now that we didn't go for the easy option.

As we stood on the hillside looking around at Besaniya, and thinking of the years of development, the problems encountered and where we had now reached with the work, we started to consider how we had been blessed. Building it all up hadn't been without problems, but prayers had been answered, dedicated and committed workers had come forward, and we now had a work which met – and exceeded – our original hopes and aims. Having seen such blessing however we had to consider if we should simply stop, or whether the correct response was to try to do more.

It wasn't practical to simply make Besaniya bigger; a lot had changed since we started this work. Besaniya was as big as a 'family' could realistically become, and we had long realised that the best way to help more children was to work with them in the community. This was the thinking which eventually led to us starting schools or placing teachers as a more effective alternative to individual sponsorship. Our aim had always been to

49

try to reach those people who were most in need – and the particular emphasis of Besaniya had always been children. Having seen the work being done by Norgrove Penny with the Uganda Orthopaedic Project, we knew something of the plight of disabled children, and began to wonder if there was anything we could do to help.

When we visited Uganda, we had the opportunity to visit Mengo, and while there we looked in on Norgrove. However, Norgrove's passion for his work was such that he didn't let visitors 'look in' and then go away. We were shown around, made aware of exactly what they were trying to do, then taken up to the classroom where Norgrove explained what he was doing and why he was doing it. It was a very convincing talk – Norgrove, had he not been a surgeon, would have made a brilliant salesman. He used scripture to present a very clear mandate for work with the disabled, and also told us more of the terrible conditions endured by children who often had what to us seemed a slight disability, but in Uganda were regarded as cursed.

At the end of the visit, Norgrove took us to a side ward where we saw a number of children who had undergone surgery the previous day. It quickly became clear how, in many cases, quite a short operation could be totally life changing for the child – and make a big difference to their whole family. Norgrove presented all this to such effect that we simply couldn't go away and forget about it. There we were at Besaniya with a beautiful site, good buildings and facilities, experienced workers, a widespread network of interested people – and here were these children who desperately needed help.

Notwithstanding all this, and the fact that the Crosses, Alan and myself were enthusiastic about doing something, we hadn't the faintest idea what to do. A significant part of our Besaniya work was sponsoring the education of individual children. We wondered about the possibility of extending this to include sponsorship of operations for children who might not otherwise be helped. This seemed a good idea, easy for us to implement and something we felt donors would respond to – but when we talked to Norgrove about it, he said he had no problem with the costs of surgery, that part of the programme was already adequately covered. He pointed out that the big problem was with rehabilitation. The surgery might take a short time (in some cases only minutes), followed by a day in hospital, but there was then the need for lengthy rehabilitation – probably averaging around three months.

There were of course several centres, notably Katalemwa, dealing with this, but they were full to capacity and more provision was needed. It would be different here; many of the children could have gone home quite soon and been brought back for outpatient treatment. But in Uganda, that was impractical. How long would a plaster cast survive in a village environment? How could travel be arranged for outpatient treatment? There would also be very little access to medical services if any problem arose. The only way was to keep the children in rehabilitation units till recovery was complete and they could return to their communities. We then wondered if a few 'low dependency' children could be accommodated at Besaniya (it always seems possible to squeeze in a few more beds there when necessary) and take them to Mengo or Katalemwa for outpatient treatment. However, Besaniya is on a steep hillside, with many steps up to the main building – not ideal for a child using crutches or a wheelchair. Also, whatever type of children were brought there it would still be desirable, if not essential, to have someone with medical skills to oversee their care. To some extent these practicalities could have been dealt with, but it would never be an ideal solution and wasn't going to have much impact on the problem.

It was clear that what was needed was a purpose built rehabilitation unit, so that is what we started to think about. This whole process had taken one day since meeting with Norgrove. Having decided something needed to be done, we saw no point in wasting time when we had the chance to discuss it together. By this time there was no question of whether we would do anything, it was a question of what we would do.

12.
WHERE AND HOW

The day after Norgrove's passionate presentation of the needs of disabled children left us convinced that we should do something, and following deliberations which quickly led to the conclusion that we should build a rehabilitation unit, Alan Clegg, the Crosses and myself stood at Besaniya looking around us, trying to decide the next step.

We were agreed on what we should do; all that remained were 'details' – such as where and how. Where could we build the unit, how could we pay for it? By this time, we were used to doing things we hadn't any experience of, so weren't particularly concerned about how we could run a rehabilitation unit! We had always found the right people in the past (or, more accurately, they found us).

First, the 'where'. We weren't going to worry about how to pay for something till we had much firmer plans. We could have considered building the rehabilitation unit somewhere other than Besaniya –ideally, close to Mengo. But that was impractical, it seemed to make much more sense to make use of facilities we already had at Besaniya. The location was far from ideal, being on a steep hillside – but against that, we had staff and facilities available there. Another major consideration was being able to bring the disabled children into the Besaniya 'family', with the opportunity for them to get to know other children. Often, a disabled child would be hidden away and have no opportunity for interaction with other children, whether through school or play. In addition to treatment of their disability, they needed to be 'socialised' and in this respect Besaniya was ideal.

We then had to decide exactly where to locate the building. The decision was effectively made for us by the need for the disabled children to have access to the Besaniya dining room, classroom, library etc, all of them housed in the main building, at the upper part of the site. Fortunately, there seemed to be enough room to the side of this building if we cut back into the hillside.

The 'how' also had to be addressed – but we had always found in the past that if we had made the right decision on what to do, then the necessary support would follow. I sometimes tire of people saying they are doing something 'in faith' – it can mean they haven't bothered to do their homework properly or are planning something ill advised. If we have done everything possible to ensure we are providing the right solution to a problem, if we have been diligent in our planning, if we do everything possible to ensure maximum value, then we have the confidence to ask for help – and to trust that the necessary help will be forthcoming. We do of course believe in doing things in faith – it's how all our work has been developed – but that goes with thoroughness and the application of high standards. I also think that our big strength in asking for help is that we can show what has already been achieved through our work with Besaniya and ECM. The Crosses knew our work well, and were so touched by the needs of the disabled that they immediately offered us help through their 'Upper Room' charity.

With this promise of help, we went ahead with planning. However, we still had no opportunity to even try to guess the cost of what we had in mind.

When I got home, and after more detailed plans were prepared, we were able to approximately estimate the cost of the building, and a donor provided the total amount. This was wonderful, because we had not asked for any money. I was asked by someone I hadn't seen for a while what we were planning next in our work. When I said we wanted to build a rehabilitation unit, they asked what it would cost – and wrote a cheque.

With this gift, and the 'Upper Room' support, we had enough not just to put up the building, but to fully equip it and also build a staff house. But that is getting too far ahead – there was a lot to think about before building could start.

13.

THE TREE

We've often made use of work teams in Uganda; from the very start, they've gone out to assist with building work and other projects. We have had a big range of ages, skills and experience, and have derived great benefit from their efforts, often completing work we couldn't otherwise afford. In turn it's our hope that it has been a valuable experience for all who took part. I think it's true to say that for many their time in Uganda has been life changing; many things were never to look the same again.

People going out as volunteers or on work teams had to face challenges, everything was new to them. Climate, culture, travel, diet, everything was very different to what they were used to. Many found it rewarding to be able to meet and deal with these challenges, and do some useful work. But the real reward came in being able to look beyond these 'practicalities' to their relationship with the people. At first, what confronts us is so much that is different. The big challenge is to look beyond that to what is the same. We've had Christians go out from many denominational backgrounds; they would be familiar with expressions like 'brothers in Christ' to describe their relationship with other believers, but beyond their own church or 'circle' for most it remained a concept, not something they were able to experience at first hand. It has meant a great deal to those who have recognised that whatever differences there are between us, and the Ugandans we are working with, there's the common bond as Christians which transcends everything else and enables there to be fellowship. This adds a completely new dimension to the experience, and even if they never get back to Africa their lives have been enriched and their faith strengthened.

When I was at Besaniya with the Crosses, a small work team arrived from Canada. They came from the Elmvale Church the Crosses attend, and John and Daisy had originally made the arrangements for them to come. However, the Crosses spend half their time in Florida and had travelled out from there – they hadn't told the team they would be in Uganda, but surprised them by appearing at Entebbe airport when the team arrived.

These volunteers were dealing with a number of tasks around Besaniya while John, Daisy, Alan and myself were discussing the possibility of building a rehabilitation unit. Having decided to go ahead, and also that it would need to be built on the same level as the main building, we went up to take a closer look at the site. It was clear that we'd have to dig back into the hillside, also that some filling would be required to raise the front of the site. There was also a water tank and some underground pipes, but that could be bypassed. The most obvious problem was a large tree, right in the middle of where we wanted to build. Bear in mind that this was the day after Norgrove had sparked our interest in doing something for disabled children, and here we were already worrying about how to remove the tree so that site preparation could begin.

Some of the older Besaniya boys would have been quite happy to fell the tree, they had experience of using the chain saw at our Nakiwate forestry project. I'm afraid I didn't have much confidence in their accuracy; there was the potential to do a lot of damage if the tree came down in the wrong direction. We did though have the work team from Canada, and we thought Canadians should know how to deal with trees. Sure enough one of them, Gary, was willing to take on the task. We all watched in anticipation as he got to work with the chainsaw, and felled the tree almost exactly as planned, with just a little damage to guttering on the dining hall roof from the branches.

Felling the tree had considerable significance for us, as we really felt we were under way. I still have a piece of the timber.

The tree served as a playground for a few days, till it was all cut up for firewood. That wasn't the end of the problem though as the stump and roots remained and gave Alan Clegg a lot of problems. They chopped it, cut it, burnt it, used chemicals to try to rot it, and I think a lot of it still remains buried underneath what is now Harriett's bedroom in the Cherub building.

Work continued to prepare the rest of the site. A great deal of digging was required, and it was clear how much easier it would be were a digger available. Alan was wakened one morning by the sound of a diesel engine, and looked out to find that someone had arranged for a Ministry of Works digger to deal with site preparation. This seemed to be the answer to the problem, but it didn't quite work out that way in practice. Anyone with experience of machinery in Uganda will know that it's rarely that simple. The digger was old and well worn, with bald tyres. Then there were the usual problems of fuel, spare parts, an inexperienced driver etc. In the end, they had to go back to digging by hand, and it was very hard ground. At least we provided a lot of employment!

14.
THE BUILDER

With work under way on the site, and also on plans, we then had to think about how 'Cherub' could be built. This project was ideal for Alan Clegg. As well as having a vision for work with the disabled, this was just the kind of thing he liked to get his teeth into. Alan seemed able to deal with all the problems of running a project in Uganda without it bothering him too much.

A lot of the previous building work at Besaniya had been carried out by a local man, Musoke, and it was to him that Alan turned now. Musoke was more than just a builder, he had considerable experience and was able to give good advice. This wasn't just on building matters, he was valuable in helping Alan deal with all kinds of cultural and other issues, and they soon became friends. Another area in which Musoke differed from other Ugandan builders was in his attitude to the quality of the work. For many Ugandans, a job would be done to a standard which was just 'good enough'. Musoke however took pride in his work, and could be relied on to complete each job to a high standard, often with his own unique touches. One of the things he liked to do, for example, was apply a decorative finish to ceilings.

Some time later, Musoke came to Ireland to act as Alan's best man when he married Sara. The reception was in Durrow Castle, which has elaborate Italianate style interior decoration. Musoke was often to be seen with his eyes turned heavenward – not in prayer, but studying the detail of the ceilings, which he also photographed.

For the Cherub building, we had started thinking of something quite small – perhaps 6 beds – but then agreed on around 10. This was Africa though; where we might design something with reasonable space around beds, open areas etc, the tendency there is to fill every last inch of space, so we ended up with a 20 bed unit, plus treatment room, accommodation for a carer and the other necessary facilities.

When I got home from Uganda, I talked to an architect friend about possible designs for a suitable building. He quickly came up with a design, and although we didn't use it, it proved valuable in stimulating our thinking about exactly what was needed. Meanwhile, Alan and Musoke were visiting Katalemwa and Mengo to look at their facilities and get advice on a suitable layout.

We soon reached agreement on what was needed in the building, but I don't think we even got as far as preparing detailed plans. With Musoke, it was usually enough to tell him what was needed, and let him get on with it. I think Alan was quite happy to work this way too. It's not our usual way of doing things here, but I've seen terrible mistakes made with buildings designed by someone outside the country which fail to take account of local needs, practice, materials and conditions. There's the climate – heat, sunlight, extreme rainfall. There's availability and quality of materials. There's local building practice – many things are done differently. There are also other factors such as the extent to which they live outside the house, whereas we live inside. In the end, there wasn't really any alternative but to leave it to Musoke to build something which met the needs. We also had to think of cost – we would have been in serious difficulty trying to put up anything other than quite a basic building.

Once the foundations were in, work proceeded rapidly. We made more money available when needed, Alan kept the materials coming, and Musoke's men worked on the building without delay. This was important; we were convinced this was the right time for this work, and were trying to generate enthusiasm among our donors. The project caught people's imagination, and there was a momentum to it. Had we lost this, as so often happens, if work slowed down it would have been very difficult to get the necessary support to run it when it was finished.

It's often the case that a building project can run out of steam when it's 90% completed, but Musoke was very involved personally, and really wanted to finish everything in good time and to a high standard. He often went to

Alan with ideas for improvements. The relationship between Alan, as project manager, and Musoke, as builder, worked so well because there was mutual trust. Alan knew that Musoke would do the work properly without constantly needing to chase him or look over his shoulder, while Musoke knew that all the materials would be provided, and that all the workers would be paid on time.

As the children in Cherub would need someone near at all times should problems arise, the building incorporated accommodation for a carer. However, we soon decided that a staff house should also be built. Of course staff could have lived outside Besaniya and come in to work, but it made so much more sense to have someone on site at all times. So, when work was well advanced Musoke was asked to start work on a house to accommodate whoever would be in charge of Cherub. This house came to be known as 'Pelican' house – all the Besaniya buildings are named after an animal or bird. Alan liked the name 'Pelican' because in folklore the Pelican gives its blood to its young, and it is the symbol for the Irish Blood Transfusion Board.

As with other building work, we agreed on the accommodation needed in the house – living room, kitchen, bathroom, three bedrooms so that guests could be accommodated – and left it to Musoke to build it. Once more, no detailed plans were necessary; no one would probably have looked at them anyway! Although we tried to build everything at minimum cost, Musoke couldn't keep his creativity fully under control, and incorporated some very decorative ceilings!

The site for Pelican is spectacular – with such a view, it would be worth a fortune here. It's at the other side of the site from Cherub, but on the same level so access is good. It looks out over Besaniya to the hills and lake beyond.

The decision to build the rehabilitation unit was taken in March; when I visited in November, the Cherub building was complete, and they were plastering the internal walls of Pelican house. Everything done to a good standard, and with costs tightly controlled. Musoke justifiably took considerable pride in what had been achieved, and seemed also to have caught the vision for what we were trying to achieve.

I know that Alan also derived great satisfaction at this point. He had gone to Uganda as 'project manager' for us, without us really having thought through what the title meant – I don't think either of us imagined anything on this scale, but Alan seemed able to happily deal with whatever came along, so long as it kept him busy.

So now we had our buildings, it was time to think very quickly what we were going to do with them.

15.

EUREKA

When the decision was taken to build a rehabilitation unit for disabled children, we then tried to think of a name – this was important, as we wanted to start right away the process of making the project more widely known and trying to generate support. The Crosses, Alan and I discussed this. Alan, being the closest we had to a poet amongst us, was coming up with the most imaginative names, but we really wanted a title which adequately described what the unit was, and the initials of which would form an easily remembered name. We were coming up with plenty of initials, but struggled to make them into any kind of a sensible name that would also have some connection to what we were doing.

We had other things to do, and couldn't spend all day worrying about a title so left it for the time being. The Crosses and I, while not forgetting about it, got on with what we were doing. Alan however wouldn't let it go and I think he continued to go through all kinds of possibilities. Then, late in the day, he had his 'eureka' moment and told us he had chosen a name. Cherub. Child Health Education and Rehabilitation Unit, Besaniya. I'm not sure where the inspiration came from. Previously we'd been thinking of titles and trying to make a word from the initials. This time, Alan did it the other way round. He'd been thinking of all kinds of words then trying to make up a title using all the letters. So it was with Cherub – he chose the name, then went on to make to full title from it. As well as being unable to fault his thinking, this was a big relief to us as we hadn't been able to come up with anything else which worked – and so 'Cherub' it was. There is some quite imaginative art work on the end of the building to illustrate the name, and the builders worked the name into the steelwork of the fence. It has gone on to become a very well known name.

16.
HARRIETT

We now had buildings, but no staff and no patients. In reality, keeping pace with all the work so far had left little time for thinking ahead. We knew that before Cherub could develop to its full potential, we would need professional staff – at the minimum a physiotherapist or nurse. We did though have other workers at Besaniya who could help, such as Fred and Mirica Kisitu, the house parents in the home, as well as other staff. They could help supervise children if the patients brought in didn't need too much care, and Besaniya is close to Mukono Health Centre where medical services were available if required. What was essential though was someone to live in Cherub with the children, in particular to deal with any problems which arose during the night.

I was glad to be there in November 2000. I had been there in March, when we took the decision to start the work and I was back in November when, from however small a beginning, Cherub made the step from being just a building to functioning as a rehabilitation unit.

All concerned were agreed that the next step was to employ a resident 'carer' for the children. There are procedures to be followed when seeking to recruit someone. We needed someone, if not with qualifications, then at least with the experience needed to care for children. So far, no problem. The difficulty lay in finding someone without family ties who could quickly leave everything and move in 'permanently' to Cherub. They also had to be willing to be there most of the time rather than having a more conventional working day.

We didn't want the recruitment to be a long process, as we could lose the momentum which the project had up to then. Our Besaniya workers knew

65

many people in the local community, and they suggested talking to Harriett Nakabuye, who was living nearby. At this time Harriett had no home of her own and was living with relatives; she was also very keen to find work locally. Harriett's story was typical of many; one of many children by a father who had a number of wives, and the family couldn't afford to send her to school. She married very young, had two children, and then her husband left, leaving Harriett to bring them up.

Harriett was approached and expressed interest. She was then asked to attend Besaniya for interview. We were now in a position we'd often been in before, and would be in again. I can't remember an occasion when we had a choice in selecting workers, usually when someone was needed we would find there was only one person available, and thankfully they usually turned out to be right for the job. Along with the Kisitus and Alan Clegg, I helped conduct the interview with Harriett, without any real idea of what I should be asking her. I think this was also a frightening experience for Harriett, but she was known to be of good character, to have useful experience, and was immediately available. It was therefore an easy decision to make, and Harriett was offered the job for a 'probationary' period to ensure she was satisfactory.

Poor Harriett had no idea what she was taking on. She certainly wanted work so accepted a job when it was offered, but Cherub was an empty building and she had no way of knowing what her job would eventually entail. As we'd often seen however, when someone is given responsibility, even for something they have no previous experience of, they rise to the challenge. So it was with Harriett who proved very capable, took pride in her work, and steadily took on more responsibility as she gained experience. Most importantly, everyone working at Besaniya has to integrate as part of a big 'family' and Harriett soon had good relationships with everyone.

From starting as an 'assistant' or 'carer' Harriett was able to progress to assistant manager when Cherub was fully operational, dealing with administration and helping with medical treatment as well as supervising the children.

17.
ANOTHER TREE

Everything now seemed to be in place to at least get Cherub started, but we needed patients. Without skilled medical staff we weren't yet ready to start accepting referrals from the Uganda Orthopaedic Project for post operative care. What we really needed were children who couldn't yet return to their own home for whatever reason, but didn't need much medical attention. Several cases were brought to our notice but unfortunately we were unable to help as they needed more specialised care. And although Cherub had been built primarily to provide rehabilitation for disabled children, we agreed that we didn't need to be too rigid about this, and could consider other cases if we thought we could help. With a completely new work, which most people knew nothing about, we weren't going to get many people coming looking for us but we did have a network of associates in our work with ECM and it was through them that the first patient was found.

Not long before starting Cherub, ECM started work on several of the more remote islands in Lake Victoria. We were fortunate in having our own boat, and workers were able to travel to the islands under Patrick's direction. The first island we worked on was Jana, and on one of his visits Patrick was shown a boy of around 12 years old, James, who had fallen out of a tree and broken his femur. There was no medical attention of any kind available on Jana, and presumably no one could afford to take James anywhere else for treatment, so he had been lying for over a week, in considerable pain, steadily getting weaker.

James was taken across the island to the boat – I understand he was transported on a bicycle! He was taken to the mainland in the ECM boat, and then to Mengo Hospital – a very difficult journey for him in his weakened condition. We were eventually to have a lot of trouble trying to convince islanders to let us take disabled children to Cherub, but there were no such problems with James – he was obviously very ill, and no one else was able to do anything.

At Mengo, the fracture was set and we agreed that he could come to Cherub for rehabilitation as it seemed he wouldn't require medical treatment there, and could be taken back to Mengo for the plaster to be removed. There then started some frantic preparations to get a bed ready, and for Harriett to move into her new accommodation.

The question of transport then arose. James was completely immobile, in an extensive plaster cast, so an 'ambulance' was necessary. Alan had the answer; he stripped the seats out of his Toyota people carrier and put a mattress on the floor. I was there when they arrived back at Cherub with James; he must have been terrified. This was such a significant event, the first patient being admitted, that everyone gathered to take pictures as he was unloaded and brought inside.

We'd made it. From an idea in March, here we were with a 'finished' work only 8 months later. There was still a long way to go, skilled staff to recruit, equipment to be installed, procedures to be established, but Cherub was now operational and an accepted part of the Uganda Orthopaedic Project. James went on to make a good recovery, and before long Cherub would be full of children of all ages. James looked so lonely as the only patient in Cherub, but it was a memorable day and I was very glad to have been there to see it. I knew it also meant a great deal to Alan.

18.

THE CROCODILE

Care in African hospitals can be very different from what we have come to expect here. Usually the hospital provides the medical care with everything else dealt with by the family – feeding, washing, bedding etc. It's a system which enables the hospitals to be run at lower cost, bringing treatment within the reach of more people, but it's not without its problems.

For a start, the hospital can become very crowded. Often it's not a case of one relative caring for the patient, the whole family may come along. A mother caring for a sick child will have her other children to think of too; they all need to be fed, so the hospital grounds can look absolutely chaotic with so many cooking fires, washing drying etc. The relatives also need somewhere to sleep, so quite a few people can sometimes occupy one hospital bed – either on it or under it. Some of these relatives have no previous knowledge of hospitals, which can cause problems. They may light cooking fires in the hospital ward. They may bring in live animals as a source of food. I know of one case elsewhere in Africa where a nurse doing a ward round was horrified to find a live crocodile tied up under a child's bed!

It would have been usual for at least the mothers to stay with children in Cherub. For a number of reasons however, we didn't want this to be the case – and it caused surprise in some quarters. Space was restricted. We could accommodate a maximum of 20 children; if their mothers stayed too, we couldn't have so many patients. The exception was for very young children, and the mothers who stayed were expected to help with the general running of Cherub. Some also needed to be trained in the methods needed to care for their children. Otherwise, we preferred not to have them around. It wasn't a problem providing food for the children, they were able to eat with all the other Besaniya children. There was washing to deal with (children, clothes, bedding) and that was sometimes chaotic until an EM work team built a separate block with better facilities. Another factor was the parents' expectations of the child. In rehabilitation it can be important to 'push' the child, get them doing things they mightn't have been capable of before. We had to be careful in Cherub about raising the parent's expectations, but equally we also have problems with parents not expecting enough of the child and not pushing them hard enough. It therefore became the norm for Cherub staff to provide all the necessary care, with a small number of mothers of very young children helping with cleaning, washing etc.

Most of those treated in Cherub are from poor families, but they are still expected to pay something towards the child's care. We obviously know that Cherub must be subsidised, we will never cover our costs from patients' fees but the running costs have been kept to a minimum and even a very modest payment from families can make a difference to the budget. But it's not just a question of trying to get back some of our costs, we want the families to feel that they are providing for their child rather than just accepting charity. Of course, no child would ever be turned away if their parents couldn't pay, nor would anyone be asked to pay more than they can realistically afford. Any charges are very small.

19.

SUSPICIONS

The Besaniya Children's Home had been in operation for 15 years before Cherub was thought of. Till then, any change had been gradual. Occasionally an older boy would leave, or there would be another admission. Every few years there might be a new member of staff. In general though it was very stable, and the children certainly weren't used to any dramatic change. Any building work undertaken was usually to accommodate more staff or children. Change was regarded with suspicion by the boys – how was it going to affect them? And of course there would be rumours, a very serious problem there. Despite having been there for a long time, it was common for some of the children to feel insecure or threatened.

They watched everything that went on. When there were visitors, or any new faces, there would be conjecture about why they were there. This was made a lot worse at times by some of the older boys who would act as 'spies', see or hear things, then add two and two together and get five. It only took one troublemaker to cause serious instability. Because of this, we tried to avoid doing anything which would create these fears. Whatever our policy on having children stay in Besaniya, it could be undermined by what another child might say – and unfortunately, they would sometimes be all too ready to listen to another child rather than to what we were telling them. We had always tried to ensure that a child never felt under threat. Certainly at times there was bad behaviour, and it had to be punished, but we tried to have all the children understand that Besaniya was their home, and they wouldn't be put out. Only in the most extreme cases did we ever look for an alternative to keeping a child in the home and even then we didn't give up responsibility for them.

It was however necessary to look at ways of making the boys

independent, steering them towards adult life and self sufficiency. With this in mind, we looked at how our small numbers of university students could be moved out to hostel accommodation to free up more spaces in the home. We little realised the problems this was going to cause, and only then saw how little thought any of them had given to their future. This started us looking at ways of involving a child in planning their future, including trying to set a time for their 'graduation' from Besaniya. None of what we did though completely solved the problem of insecurity. If we encouraged a student to move out, or an older boy to get a job, soon a number of others would be complaining to all and sundry that we were trying to force them out too, when we had no intention whatsoever of doing so.

It was against this background that work started on Cherub. The work was done on the upper part of the site, away from the houses, so there was minimal disruption to day to day life in the home – but what the children saw was major change taking place when things had remained the same for years. We did our best to explain to them. One or two saw it as a good idea that we would help more children; others quickly started spreading stories that we wanted them out so that Besaniya would become some kind of hospital. We tried our best to involve them in the work, but the fears remained. We could have built Cherub somewhere else, but wanted it within Besaniya for a number of reasons. It would avoid duplication of services, enable better use to be made of Besaniya facilities, but most of all the disabled children would be coming into a 'family' and we hoped eventually the Besaniya children would relate well to the children brought in for rehabilitation.

Over time, some of the fears were replaced by curiosity. The children had inevitably very little understanding of disability, as attitudes were such that they would rarely come in contact with it, and to some extent wouldn't even have been aware of its existence. They had a lot to learn. We wanted to change attitudes to the disabled, and the first place we began to see this happen was with the Besaniya children. Although there was the stigma attached to disability, it was soon clear that children there paid very little attention to appearance. It didn't seem to matter what someone looked like, what really mattered was what they were capable of. If they couldn't play with them, no one was particularly interested. Certainly someone who was relatively immobile or confined to bed was of no interest whatsoever. It was also clear that for most of the boys, unless there was something in it for them, they weren't interested in helping. Many of them played with the Cherub children when they were able to get out and about, but after the initial curiosity few bothered to visit the unit. Once it became clear Cherub wasn't a threat, they simply ignored it. We had hoped the children would have taken a greater interest, and shown a desire to help others, but it didn't really happen. There were a few exceptions , one or two starting to help on a regular basis – and in fact they went on to become very useful even if at times it was hard to tell what their motives were. Did they want to help, or was this an alternative to studying or doing homework? Eventually though several of the boys expressed a desire to train as nurses, physiotherapists or doctors, and we have been supporting one boy through medical school. Another, the most regular helper in Cherub, has now started nursing training.

Five years on, Cherub is now fully integrated into Besaniya, it is simply taken for granted. Most of the boys pay very little attention to it, but it does seem that for children there is very little consciousness of disability, the problem is with adults. The children are just accepted as playmates, seemingly regardless of appearances. It is often frightening though to see the games played by children with plasters or other appliances – very little allowance is made.

For the Cherub children, I think there have been substantial benefits in having them in Besaniya. In the past they probably haven't had the opportunity to mix with other children, and consequently have been made to feel different. Having other children treat them as normal has made a big difference and their development can be very rapid. From being shy and withdrawn, they quickly become much more outgoing and confident. Their recovery is certainly speeded by all the exercise and outdoor activity.

20.

THE PHYSIO

With Cherub under way, there was a real urgency to find someone medically qualified to take charge. With Harriett there, and the health centre nearby, it was possible to care for recovering children – but not in the way we'd originally envisaged. It's not always easy to find someone prepared to leave everything and go off to work in Africa for a few years, and even for those willing to go, preparations can take some time. We had a few 'false starts', people we hoped would go, but couldn't, or ones who might have been willing but didn't seem to be the person we wanted, for whatever reason.

It is always a big concern sending someone out. They must be sufficiently capable and confident to take control of a situation very different from what they are used to, but must also be prepared to live as part of the Besaniya family and place themselves under authority. A 'dominant' personality can easily damage relationships or undermine confidence.

We seemed to need either a nurse or physiotherapist, and weren't sure which would be most suitable – in fact I think we would have accepted either. A physiotherapist would be ideal for dealing with assessment of disability, and post operative care and rehabilitation. However, there were medical needs which a nurse could deal with, although the children would have needed to go elsewhere for physio if we couldn't find one locally. We couldn't afford both, so had to compromise. The expert view was that a physiotherapist would be most suitable, so that is what we tried to find, though we would still have settled for an experienced nurse, and the Cherub intake would have been chosen to suit that.

There was no possibility at that time of finding a Ugandan physiotherapist, there were few of them around. Also, particularly to start with, we preferred to send someone from here. We had been fortunate in being given the necessary funds to build Cherub, but now needed to build up a support base to keep it all running, and having someone from here would help greatly. At that time, few people in Uganda would have recognised the need for physiotherapy so it was a profession few followed. Medical treatment was costly for most people; as soon as someone was well enough to leave hospital they would be gone, and it was extremely difficult to persuade anyone to return for what they saw as the 'option' of physiotherapy.

One of the few physiotherapists we knew was Florence Mawhinney. We knew she had an interest in serving overseas, so asked if she would consider working in Cherub. However, Florence's experience was all with adults and she didn't want to make the switch to working with children. We thought that was the end of that, and continued to look elsewhere- with conspicuous lack of success. Fortunately, Florence continued to think about Cherub and one day we got a message to say that she would be interested. We made it clear that as the professional Florence would be totally in control of the patients admitted and the type of work undertaken, and she agreed to go for two years. She made all her preparations as quickly as possible, and was ready to go to Uganda in April 2001.

There was also the matter of how to pay her. Florence hadn't stipulated any requirements for a 'salary', but we had to pay her something and we didn't have very much. If we paid her even a modest allowance, we wouldn't have much left for running costs – and there was still equipment to buy. Fortunately APSO, the Dublin based and government funded agency which helped support personnel overseas, was willing to help and not only provided a generous allowance, but responded very quickly when we sought their help. They have given us a lot of help over the years which has meant a great deal to us.

Florence had a lot to deal with when she got to Cherub; as well as developing relationships with all those she would live and work with, she had to establish working procedures for the unit. Instead of just being a physiotherapist she had to become a manager – which she did very effectively. She was soon working very closely with Norgrove Penny at

Mengo and with Katalemwa, which served as a referral centre and Cherub's main link with the Uganda Orthopaedic Project.

There was no shortage of patients, and the numbers in Cherub quickly built up. As people came to know of the work, attitudes began to change and more children were brought for Florence to see. Cherub was there to deal with a particular range of disability but when clinics were run, the general shortage of medical facilities meant that all kinds of patients wanted to be seen. Particularly with rural clinics, it was very difficult to simply refuse to help and the work of Cherub started to become much wider.

Florence was the person who got Cherub properly under way, finding what everyone involved was capable of, determining policy, deciding on the type of work which could be undertaken, assessing and referring children for surgery or appropriate treatment, and also trying hard to do something to help those patients who fell outside the Cherub criteria. From being a new facility with no clear policy or direction, Cherub now was being run professionally, and the difference could be clearly seen. This gave people confidence – and the nature of the work was such that children and parents had to put a lot of trust in us. How it all appeared to them was therefore very important.

Another major consideration was that Florence was able to send us back detailed reports of case histories which we could use to encourage further support. We had fears also about how much it would cost to run Cherub, but we needn't have worried as it turned out to be very cost effective and functioned on a modest budget.

We had seen a number of big steps taken – deciding to go ahead, starting work on the building, being given funds, seeing the buildings finished, admitting the first patient etc. Soon there was another very big step when we were able to look at the first 'before' and 'after' pictures of children helped, and see the clear evidence of the difference Cherub had made. Not only did a child have a disability treated, perhaps enabling them to walk for the first time; they would no longer be an outcast and could look forward to doing all the things 'normal' children did. A Ugandan child didn't seem to worry about what disability meant to their appearance. What they usually wanted above all else was to be able to go to school.

Florence writes:

November 2001:

"By the time I had arrived in Cherub in April 2001 one patient had already been and gone. There were also six overflows from Katalemwa to get me started. Since April I have assessed 134 children. 47 were admitted to Cherub and 33 of these were surgical cases. The average length of stay is approximately 13 weeks. A further 41 cases were cerebral palsy children, many of whom come to Cherub's weekly cerebral palsy clinic. 15 children are currently waiting for treatment, primarily surgery, and the remaining 31 cases were either seen as outpatients at Cherub or a rural clinic. A rural clinic is held in Kisogo (15 miles away). Three other local clinics have been held in other areas, with more planned.

"Cherub has taken off. I am satisfied that it is achieving its intended purpose, and Dr Penny is also very happy with the work. I have employed a young local nurse to supervise Cherub at the weekends to relieve Harriett and myself."

February 2002:

"Saidi continues to battle on with good and bad days, but is now without plaster of Paris for the first time in about 2 years. He must wear a special boot though as the bone is still unstable but we continue to leave him in God's hands. My latest little character is a tiny 7 year old with bilateral club feet, abandoned by his parents probably because they assumed he was cursed. He was brought to us by a local villager. Paul is the size of a 3 year old because of malnourishment, and he also has TB so cannot have surgery yet. I have been stretching his feet with plaster of paris in preparation for surgery but the results have been so good he may not require surgery after all. When he first came he hardly spoke and was not toilet trained. We all assumed he had mental problems but is now recognised as one of the most intelligent children we have. We hope to track down his parents and see if they will accept him back when they see he is normal after all, but the TB medication takes 8 months to complete."

17th June 2002:

"Saidi has made great progress, and was able to go home for two weeks. He hadn't been home for two years, during which his father had moved several times. However, he was tracked down and the reunion eventually made. As a spectator, I had to laugh as Harriett struggled to relay her list of instructions regarding Saidi's care to his non-Luganda speaking father, with the boda boda man (motorcycle taxi driver) translating and adding his own ideas to the list of fruit and vegetables he needed. He has now returned to Cherub revitalised. Paul, the malnourished child with TB and club feet, seems to have more insight than many 15 year olds, and has something to say on every issue. It is hard to believe that 8 months ago we thought he was brain damaged. He provides us all with great entertainment and will be sadly missed. He will be leaving walking normally, and our prayer is that his own family will now accept him and give him the love and affection he was quite obviously bereft of all his life.

"Cherub is making a difference. I wish you could all come and see for yourself. Let me encourage you to never underestimate the power of simple, practical and even short but sincere prayers. This is not work a few people over in Uganda are doing. I see it as work we are all doing together and God will reward each of us for sacrificing whatever time, money or talents we can."

7th November 2002:

"Saidi went home last week, and will return in February for assessment to see if his new bone is strong enough for further surgery to lengthen it. He is now walking with one crutch. At one time Dr Penny talked about amputation, but we praise God it didn't come to that. He has changed since he came here, and is more outgoing and very responsible.

"Susan Nansombe is an 11 year old girl who has been with us since March. She too has a very aggressive multiple site osteomyelitis. She came with her tibia bone exposed completely. This bone was removed in the first of a series of operations and to our surgeon's amazement a new tibia has started to grow. She has other knee and ankle problems which will be addressed in time but currently needs time for the bone to strengthen, physio to mobilise the knee, and dressings for the big hole in her foot. She is a strong girl and determined to do her exercises every day.

"Edith Bagambe, 11, has also been with us since March. She has severe brittle bone disease in her lower limbs; the deformities in her legs were very severe and difficult to treat. Her legs are not perfect, but much better than before.

"Pascal Nsekanaba, a bright 17 year old who suffered polio in his right foot when very young, has had two surgeries so far and will be in plaster till January. He's now very happy with his foot. He will need a splint, but will be able to wear shoes. The stigma that he felt was probably his biggest concern; it has changed his life and he is so grateful.

"Peter Silingi is a 13 year old boy with severe polio affecting his legs above and below the knee so he could only get around on his hands and knees. He had surgery to release the contractures. Once equipped with callipers, he will walk upright for the first time in years.

"Robinah Namulini, 15 years old. Yet another case of multiple site osteomyelitis. She has just had her first surgery with the usual horrendous wounds which no longer shock Harriett or myself. She will hopefully make a full recovery."

December 2002:

"Since opening its doors Cherub has assessed 277 children to date (November 2002). 102 have been admitted and the rest have either attended as outpatients, are awaiting further treatment, have failed to re-attend or only required a one off consultation. The most common conditions seen are osteomyelitis (bone infection) with all the associated complications, club feet, post injection paralysis, polio, congenital and acquired bone deformities and cerebral palsy. We are getting the most severe cases that you simply would never see in the west mainly because the majority of families are very poor so are unwilling to take the child for treatment when the condition is in its early stages. This is why the length of stay can often be very prolonged, as many require more than one surgical procedure before they are ready for discharge. For some, Cherub has been a life saver. The ages have ranged from newly borns to 19 years and we have had good success with all.

"We are known to the health authorities and I recently attended a meeting for Mukono District specifically about sensitising the community to club feet and how it should be treated. Cherub was identified as one of only two centres where there are Ponsetti (the treatment of choice) trained personnel who can deal with the problem in newly borns and we are the only unit who can deal with the problem if the neglected club foot requires surgery. These links are vital if we are to work together to eradicate the neglected club foot in Uganda. They will also be using the statistics I have gathered on other preventable disabilities such as post injection paralysis to help address this unnecessary disability.

"Other field workers have come to know about Cherub, including many pastors and through these contacts I have been able to do some clinics. This is useful because I can rely on these contacts to help me with follow up of their children.

"The vision for Cherub was clearly divinely inspired. At the outset all of us involved were unsure of what exactly Cherub's role would be but it has developed so naturally and smoothly we are in no doubt that God has been at work through us, setting everything in place so as to meet the needs of many children. It has a definite role to play in the lives of Ugandan children and has already changed many.

"I have enjoyed my time immensely and feel blessed to have been asked to come here. The children are a joy to work with and the Besaniya family is a joy to be part of."

21.

THE PRESIDENT

My first trip to Uganda was in 1984. Over the next 20 years I've made many more visits, usually travelling out at least once a year for varying periods of time. I have so many memories of these visits, many of which went past in a blur. It's been such a rich experience but I have seen so much, and met so many people, that it's hard to 'order' all these recollections. My memories tend to be in a series of 'snapshots' of notable or significant events – arriving for the first time at Entebbe, first sight of the Nile, seeing a child dying from Aids, my first Ugandan thunderstorm, my first journey to the islands, as well as memories of my first meetings with a number of individuals who would become important to our work.

One such unforgettable moment came on 24th October 2001 when I stood at Besaniya phoning home to tell Hazel about the official opening of Cherub, and listening to the departing helicopters carrying the Irish president and other VIPs. The previous days had been so hectic it was only now that it was sinking in, and I was able to take stock of all that had happened since we stood on the hillside and talked about building the rehabilitation unit. I also thought back 20 years to the time a number of us stood on the same hillside (at that time bare) and discussed the building of Besaniya Children's Home. As I looked around, I tried to see beyond all the attractive buildings, and the landscaped site now looking so mature with all its trees etc, to the large numbers of people who had now been touched by this work. How blessed we were to have seen our dreams and ideas become reality.

The first patient was admitted to Cherub in November 2000. Florence arrived there in April 2001 and this was the beginning of Cherub's development as an integral part of the Uganda Orthopaedic Project. Since then Cherub had continued to operate to capacity, but occasionally someone would suggest having an official opening. Our first reaction was not to worry too much about it, but then we began to think that the attendant publicity could be useful for Cherub. We wanted as many people as possible to know about it so that we could try to change attitudes to the disabled. It was still some time though till we got round to doing something about it.

During 2001 Alan Clegg heard that the Irish president Mary McAleese planned to visit East Africa. The Irish ambassador talked to Alan about this; the president was to visit a number of projects with Irish connections, and the ambassador wanted to add Besaniya to the list. We were delighted as we had received generous help in the past through Irish government agencies. As we discussed the presidential visit the subject of an official opening for Cherub came up and we wondered if Mary McAleese would do this. Alan went along and asked the ambassador – from start to finish the staff of the embassy couldn't have been more supportive. Soon, word came back that the president was willing to perform the opening ceremony and a period of frantic planning started. We wanted to be clear about what we wanted from the event, and to make sure we got maximum advantage from it.

There was a lot of excitement when news of what was planned became known. Few people there knew anything about Mary McAleese, but the fact of a president, any president, visiting was a major event and a big boost for the entire local community. There were those at Besaniya though who refused to believe that a woman could be a president!

Africare is primarily an evangelical protestant organisation based in N Ireland so before long politics reared its head, with questions asked about the possible repercussions of having the Irish president perform the opening. For myself, and I must say for everyone else, without exception, who I discussed it with, this was not an issue. It was not a political visit. If the Irish president was happy to work with us, then we were happy to work with them. I think everyone took the visit at face value and accepted it as an endorsement of what we had been doing there. We had also been happy with any opportunity to work in co operation with other Irish based agencies, and Cherub had opened up new possibilities for working with others. We are only too pleased that others are willing to work with us and co operate with us; we have certainly never felt any need to compromise our own beliefs by working with others. We actively encouraged anyone coming in contact with disabled children to make referrals to us, and there were also opportunities to jointly organise clinics. Co operation has always been beneficial to our work, enabling us to do collectively what we couldn't have done alone.

We knew some of the other projects the president intended to visit. Inevitably, her visit was seen as a big event and large celebrations were planned with big crowds expected to attend. At first we looked at effectively throwing open Besaniya to the local community, inviting large numbers of guests, but then we started to think more carefully about how the official opening could be of most benefit to us. We decided it would be much better to keep the numbers down. We'd still be able to generate widespread publicity but by keeping the numbers small it would be a much more special event for our own workers. We wanted their efforts to be recognised as they were the ones making Cherub possible. We therefore only invited church or community representatives if they meant something to our work and we'd good reason to have them there.

I was due to travel to Uganda anyway, so was able to time my visit to coincide with the Cherub opening. I travelled out with Florence's mother Ella, and Fred Picking who for years had been helping me with medical equipment and wanted to visit for himself. Fred and I took the opportunity to visit Mengo and Kiwoko hospitals and give whatever help we could with medical equipment – but most of our time was taken up at Besaniya, with intensive preparations for the big event. I was happy to leave planning to others, in particular Alan who was working closely with the embassy staff. My main concern was to get my speech written, but I soon found out more was required of me.

When I'm in Uganda I prefer to keep a low profile. Because I am seen as the 'boss' certain things are expected of me but rather than attending meetings etc, I'm much happier getting my hands dirty working on something. But in the week preceding the Cherub opening there were events to attend. This involved 'dressing up' which wasn't easy, as I'd gone to Uganda prepared for work.

First event was a reception for Mary McAleese in the Sheraton Hotel in Kampala. A highlight of the evening was the Irish ambassador putting his job in jeopardy by introducing the president as Mary Robinson, her predecessor! This was my first opportunity to meet the Irish president, and we were all very warmly received. It was a very enjoyable evening with an opportunity to meet personnel from other projects in different parts of the country. We seek to maximise any opportunity open to us, so these were much more than social events. We were always looking for opportunities to promote our work, to meet people who might be helpful to us in some way, or to find out more about what other people were doing and look for chances for co operation.

The next event was a big one, as I had an invitation to attend a state dinner hosted by the president of Uganda, Yoweri Museveni, to welcome Mary McAleese. This was quite an occasion with an excellent meal, bands playing in the gallery etc. I shared a table with a number of politicians and diplomats, none of whom I knew. But before long, what had started out as a bit of an ordeal turned into a very enjoyable evening and I was pleased to find out how many Christians were present, and how many genuinely had an interest in the needs of children.

22.
WHERE ARE THE TEA BAGS?

Behind the scenes at Besaniya, preparations went on for the opening, with excitement building. The grounds had never looked better; everyone had taken a lot of care with the appearance of Besaniya, and it was paying off now. The president's visit was the spur to try to deal with any outstanding problems, and everything was brought up to an impressive standard. If we were to get maximum benefit from the publicity surrounding the opening, we at least had to look as if we knew what we were doing. Also, the president's visit wouldn't be confined to Cherub, she would also be seeing around the home. A lot of paint was used in a very short period.

The events surrounding the opening were carefully planned. The president was to unveil a plaque on the Cherub verandah, and this was provided by the Irish embassy. We fixed it in place and then tried to arrange a curtain which Mary McAleese could pull back when performing the official opening. Using whatever materials were to hand a number of people rigged a curtain on a rail which could be pulled back by a string. The finishing touch was taking the handle from one of the toilet cisterns and attaching it to the string. We had a full rehearsal with Ella Mawhinney standing in for Mary McAleese; when she pulled the handle to draw back the curtain and uncover the plaque, a tape recorder could be heard playing the sound of a toilet flushing. Thankfully, this wasn't repeated at the 'real' event.

The road approaching Besaniya was in a worse state than I'd ever seen it, but the impending visit sparked a flurry of activity and just in time repairs were completed. Because Besaniya is on a hillside, the last stretch of road up the hill is always a problem, suffering a lot of damage from heavy rain. The president's party were to arrive by road and leave by helicopter, but there was nowhere at Besaniya to land them so the playing fields at the bottom of the hill, adjoining the university and local school, were used. The children there had never seen anything like it, and I don't think any useful work could be done for the rest of the day.

Early on the morning of the big event, military personnel started to arrive to deal with security. They had also made a number of preliminary visits. There were soldiers with rifles, machine guns, rocket launchers, sniffer dogs. We were all turned out of the houses and a thorough search followed. They also set up a metal detecting arch similar to those seen at airports for everyone to walk through. This was on the upper path to Cherub, so most people used the lower path and steps to avoid queuing to go through it.

There was a strong media presence too, with Ugandan and Irish television and a number of newspapers. We had some material prepared for them and hoped that whatever was reported was accurate. I didn't see much of the newspaper coverage, but was very pleased with the way Cherub was portrayed on television in Ireland and Uganda. A number of the reporters seemed genuinely interested in what we were doing.

We continued to wonder, in spite of all our preparations, what could go wrong or what had been forgotten about. When the president's party arrived, instead of being directed to park where we had planned, once the passengers were out they parked on the path down to the children's houses, blocking it, which meant that when the president was taken around the home, everyone had to walk down the storm drain; thankfully it wasn't raining.

There was a reception line to meet the presidential party. Alan welcomed the president to Besaniya, and then I started to introduce her to the line of VIP guests. Unfortunately Alan and I then realised that there were people there, local politicians etc, who we didn't know. The first person I introduced the president to was the Archbishop of Uganda, he thankfully then took over and introduced her to the rest of the line.

Florence showed Mary McAleese around Cherub, where she chatted to Harriett and a number of the children. I was pleased to see the time the journalists were taking to talk to the children – although what the children made of it all I can't imagine, most were from village backgrounds and didn't speak English. I suppose they appreciated that something important was happening, and in Uganda any kind of party is associated with food so they were probably anticipating something extra later.

We had planned that the speeches would take place in the Besaniya dining room, and a big effort had gone into rounding up the best furniture, crockery etc. The plaque to be unveiled was outside on the Cherub verandah however, and a decision was quickly taken to make the speeches from there despite the increased security concerns. I had to make my speech first. I had spent days writing a speech, trying to compress all I wanted to say about the establishment and development of Besaniya and Cherub into the time available. When I'd done that, it started to read like a lecture or history lesson, so I abandoned it and decided instead to tell the story of one child to illustrate the impact of Cherub.

"Imagine a child who has never seen the sunlight for five years; who has been hidden in a corner of a hut because he is believed to be cursed; whose bones are so terribly diseased that he's described by the first doctor to see him as the "living dead." In a very short time he would have been dead.

"Then one day visitors came to his village. They looked important, arriving in a big four wheel drive vehicle. Normally they would have been expected to visit the important people in the village to introduce themselves, but these visitors were busy people, they hadn't time to spend on the usual formalities. Instead, they went straight to the hut where the little child was hidden. They drove past the so-called important people, straight to the little child who was believed to be cursed and they took him away.

"Imagine the impact on the whole community when, after a series of operations and lengthy rehabilitation, that little child is able to walk unaided back into the village. I can conceive of no better example of how Christ himself would have behaved in such circumstances.

"It is no good being judgmental, or blaming the child's parents or the local community. There is fear and there is a lack of knowledge. Our work is intended to open people's minds to the needs of the disabled. Indeed, the response to our clinics, the number of children being brought by parents to help them, shows how much the situation is changing.

"It's my job to find the necessary support to keep the entire work going; in fact I have become a beggar. So my thought, when there is an event like this with our distinguished visitors, is, what's in it for us?

"For me, having the president here is recognition of the efforts of everyone involved. We are a very small organisation; what you see around you represents years of struggle by all our workers, both past and present, and also loyalty from the donors who have stood by us. I especially want to mention the help we have received from Ireland through APSO, enabling us to keep our workers here when we couldn't afford to do so by ourselves; also those donors who have helped with the new development, but who through ill health are unable to attend. I hope and pray that everyone involved, from the local people through to our workers and donors, will be able to take great encouragement from what they see here and will redouble their efforts to address the needs of those who most desperately need our help."

The president then spoke, and it was clear she had been thoroughly briefed and understood exactly what we were doing. We had planned this as a day for our workers, and they were impressed that the president had taken the trouble to find out what we were doing. I was also impressed to see that she spoke without notes apart from a few headings on a piece of paper. The plaque was then unveiled and thankfully the curtain and string worked as intended.

There then followed a quick panic. The plan was to have a cup of tea – in fact, she said she could "murder a cup of tea" – and this should have been ready when she and her husband went into the dining room. Big pots of Uganda tea had been prepared for everyone else, but the tea bags Alan had bought for the president, and should have been in Pelican House, couldn't be found. With minutes to spare, Fred and Ella saved the day, quickly making the tea when the tea bags were found in Alan's house. So much for trying to ensure everything went smoothly so that it looked like we knew what we were doing! Compared to all the things which could have gone wrong, I think we got off lightly!

Thankfully despite a busy schedule the visit wasn't rushed, and the president took time to speak to all our workers – this was really appreciated, and she also made a big impression with her recall of names of the people she had been introduced to. She saw around some of our facilities including the classroom, and also went into one of the boys houses. We felt that it had all been very worthwhile, a big encouragement to our workers, and recognition of all their efforts, and a lot of valuable publicity which will help as we strive to change attitudes to the disabled.

Of course we couldn't expect everything to go perfectly, and we then had one last 'hiccup'. When the president had gone we realised we'd forgotten to present her with the gift we had for her, a batik (picture on fabric) of the home. We were able to take it to the Sheraton Hotel where the visitors were staying. The party at Besaniya went on for the rest of the day, with everyone relaxing and suitably relieved that it had gone well.

23.

SAM

By the time Cherub was operational, Alan Clegg had reached the end of the time he'd agreed to do with us in Uganda. He was willing to stay on for longer as we still needed him, but other problems were brewing which would affect this. Although Fred and Mirica Kisitu were serving as house parents at Besaniya, and Alan's role should really have been confined to projects and other work on Africare's behalf, as we had feared everyone there viewed him as being in overall control and too many problems were being passed to him to sort out. I wouldn't say that this was any one person's fault, it was more a case of the prevailing attitude. When Alan was there representing Africare, others were all too ready to avoid making decisions. This left Alan to deal with exactly the kind of responsibilities he'd said he didn't want when he went out.

Because of all this, we had to think of major changes at Besaniya. Alan agreed to stay on for longer, taking overall control until we could make other arrangements, and we brought forward the retirement date for the Kisitus. This was a very demanding time for Alan; he thought his work was done with the completion of Cherub, yet here he was now having to take full responsibility for running a children's home – and in particular deal with some of the older children who were causing us problems. I'm afraid in such circumstances it's all too easy for some people to take advantage of the situation, and Alan had plenty of work to do to keep everything running smoothly.

There was now an added factor: Alan wanted to get married. We were delighted with this news, having almost given up hope of it ever happening. He had been corresponding with a South African, Sara, and had been able to visit her. The relationship blossomed, and Alan was once more planning for a very unexpected future. To his credit, he was willing to stay with us till alternative arrangements could be made before making his own plans – and this after he had already worked much longer than he'd agreed to, and taken on responsibilities he had explicitly stated he didn't want at the time of his appointment.

We were now in a difficult position. I think we might, without too much difficulty, have found a suitable couple to replace the Kisitus, perhaps from among the ECM associates. There was though the complication that the diocese regarded the house parents as a church appointment, although my view was that Africare had interviewed, approved and paid the Kisitus from the very start. We then also needed to replace Alan; the job of house parents, and of representing Africare, were different positions. We then wondered if someone could be found to do both, taking another step on the road to handing over more responsibility. There was only one name we could think of, and other people came up with the same name. That was Sam Mutumba, a teacher from Luweero; his wife Mary was also a teacher, and we could see they had the experience and skills not just to run Besaniya, but to act for Africare. Both were however already working, were nearing retirement, and were making their own plans for the future.

Sam had been known to us for many years. He was active in the church in Luweero, and came to our attention when we had a work team there in 1989. Having seen his potential, he was asked to join ECM as a part time worker, along with our first ECM employee Patrick Wakkonyi. This proved a very significant appointment for ECM. Patrick is a pioneer, a visionary, and a very strong motivator. Sam, with his depth of experience, is a very clear strategic thinker, and together they made a very strong team. The work of ECM grew rapidly with missions, training programmes, new churches established, and a widespread network of associate workers built up. As well as whatever plans Sam and Mary had for their own future, Sam was deeply committed to the work of ECM, and we knew he would be very reluctant to leave it or to in any way reduce his involvement. Nevertheless, he really was the only person we could think of as being capable for the job.

I phoned Sam to talk to him about working at Besaniya. By now, mobile phones were everywhere in Uganda, and we were into an era of much easier communications. However, up to then I'd had very little direct contact with Sam. ECM functioned very effectively with its own local committee, and as long as I received occasional reports we transferred out the monthly budget and left them to it. Sam then wouldn't have been expecting me to phone him. When I spoke to him, he was on a bus returning to his home outside Luweero. I told him why I was ringing, and asked if he and Mary would work for us at Besaniya. This must have come as quite a shock, but he simply said he wanted to speak to Mary, and they would pray about it.

When I next rang Sam, he told me they accepted it as a call from God. Sam had asked nothing about what the job would entail, how long we wanted them for, how much they would be paid, whether there would be a contract. Yet they were willing to give up the security of their teaching jobs, put all their own plans on hold, and move to Besaniya to take on a job they knew little about. All this simply confirmed that we'd made the right choice.

Sam and Mary's acceptance now let other people get on with their own plans. The Kisitus moved out; while working for us, we had supported Fred in his training for the ministry, so now he took charge of a number of churches for the Church of Uganda while Mirica looked for a teaching job. Alan was able to make plans for his wedding, which would take place in Ireland. I remember Alan asking to be formally released from his obligations to Africare, which said a lot about the type of person he is. By that time he had gone far beyond what he'd agreed to, and I certainly didn't see him as having any remaining obligation to us. Despite all the problems and stress we caused him, we've been able to remain friends, and it was wonderful to be able to stay with Alan and Sara in their home in South Africa. It meant a lot to Alan to be able to see Cherub through to fruition. He has many friends at Besaniya, and still visits from time to time, as well as regularly phoning for news.

Sam and Mary knew we needed them urgently. Sam was able to come first, with Mary following some weeks later. They knew the importance of getting off to a good start, and I was impressed by their thoroughness in visiting all the schools, getting to know as much as possible about all the Besaniya children, and those on the external sponsorship programme. They had only been there a short time when Sam sent us proposals for all he intended to do. Both he and Mary gave themselves fully to the work, being not just effective administrators or managers, but caring parents to the children while also exercising the firmness needed to keep everything under proper control.

We still hadn't a job description for them. They were much more than house parents, and I needed any job title to reflect this. We settled on 'Field Director' for Sam, as he had to deal with wider issues for us while Mary dealt primarily with Besaniya. We little realised then just how central to our work Sam would very soon become. When he moved into Besaniya, I spoke to him on the phone and said that I was giving him authority to make decisions. All he said was "thank you for the confidence", and got on with the job.

Once more we had the right person at the right time. The growth of the work meant we had to shift the decision making to Uganda, and so we took another significant step forward. This wasn't initially understood by everyone. Some regarded this as 'temporary' and were still waiting for us to send someone else out. Others saw it as 'Africanisation', thinking we'd handed over to local control, but that wasn't the case either – Sam was our employee, and Africare remained fully responsible for all the work.

I think our biggest concern with Sam and Mary has been the amount of work they take on. I wanted their wisdom and experience, without expecting them to try to do everything themselves, but they have both put an enormous effort into what they do. Because Sam's responsibilities for us are much wider than just Besaniya, I don't think many people there realise how much he does. Of course, Cherub depends very much on Besaniya, and on Sam's overall leadership. Thankfully Sam and Mary recognise the value of what is being done there and have been very supportive.

It has been a delight to have Sam and Mary in N Ireland with us, and I hope they'll be back. Through coming here, and through the work teams we've had visit Uganda, they have made many friends.

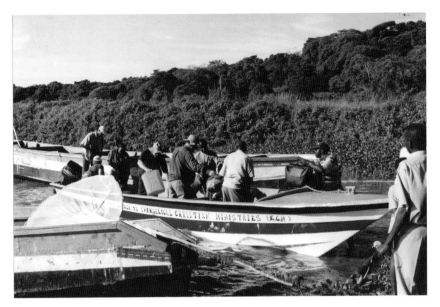

Unloading ECM boat

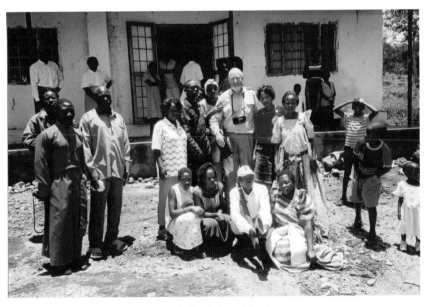

At Kisaba, Bukasa island

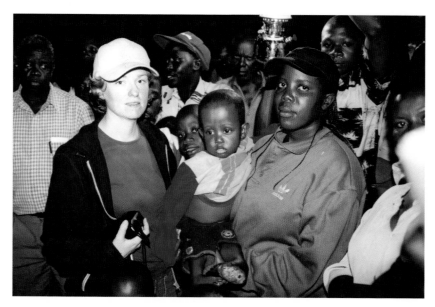

Denise Kane at Kisaba, note child's foot

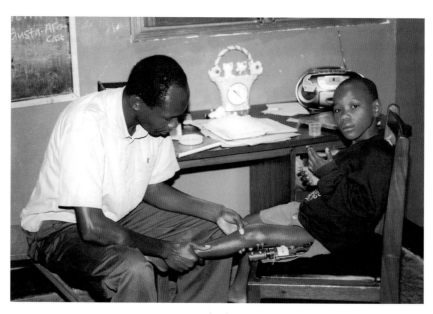

Paul Ochen

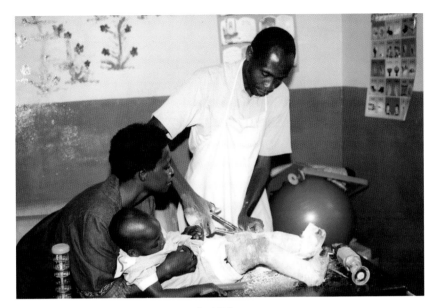

Paul Ochen

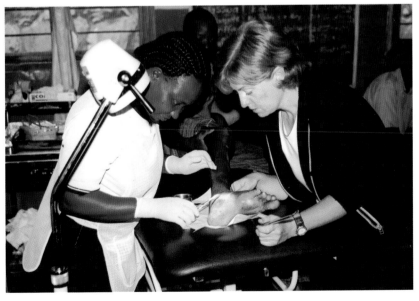

Harriet and Denise

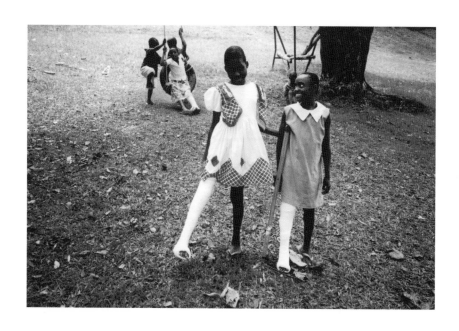

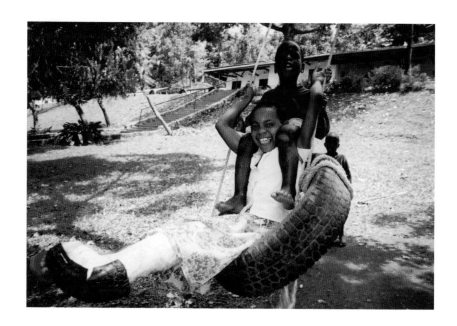

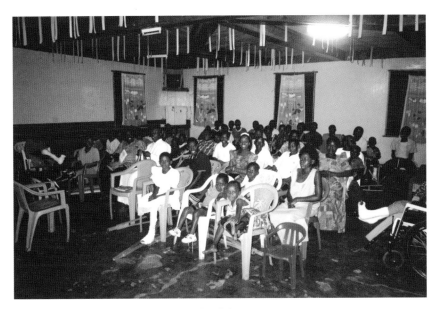

Besaniya dining room

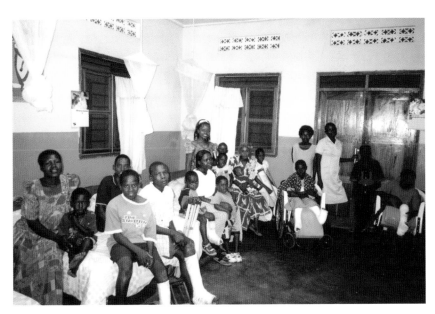

Cherub main ward

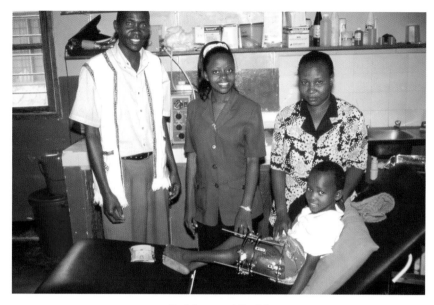

Paul, Joyce and Harriet

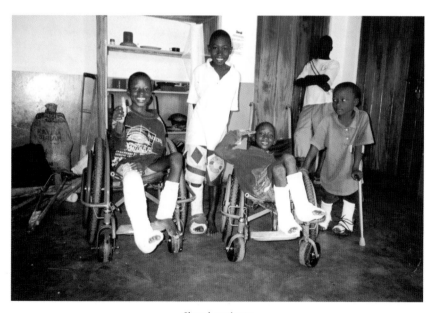

Cherub patients

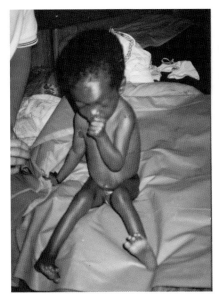
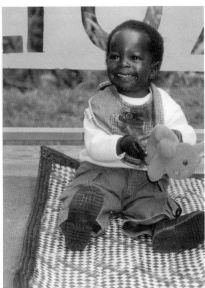

Fred Kimera, 2, before and after

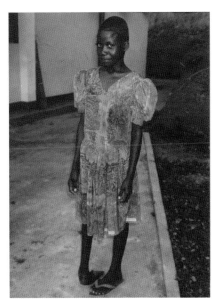
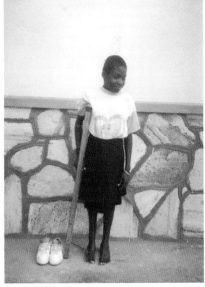

Grace Nabagala, 11, before and after

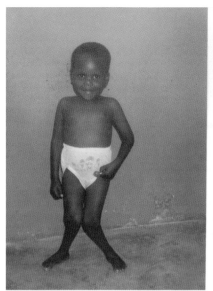
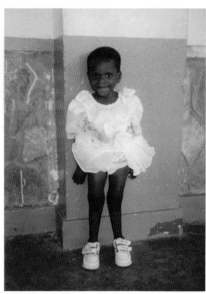

Angela Nakabuyo,7, before and after

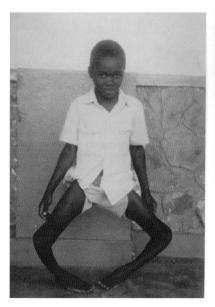
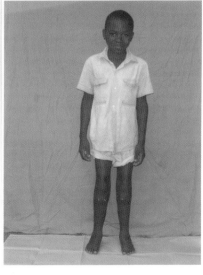

Semulya Emmanuel, 12, before and after

24.
STAFF CHANGES

It's a constant problem finding replacements for workers who leave. Florence had agreed to work for us for two years, so we were able to get Cherub properly established, but before long we had to start thinking about who could replace her. We had at one time met a Canadian physiotherapist called Danielle Mondor, when she was working with Norgrove Penny at Mengo. She had gone there I think for six months and before leaving was able to visit Cherub, around August 2000, although building wasn't completed at that stage. I met with Danielle in London when she was on her way back to Canada, and we talked then about the possibility of her working in Cherub – but the timing wasn't right, she had other commitments in Canada, and we eventually recruited Florence.

We kept in touch with Danielle, and around a year later heard that she might be interested in working for a year in Cherub. It's not always ideal having people go there for short periods of a year or two. In some ways we would have preferred someone willing to commit themselves for a much longer period. However, we had to work with what was available; also Cherub was a developing work and we weren't clear what the future might hold, so perhaps in the circumstances it was best not to try to plan too far ahead. We still had a great deal to learn.

We knew Danielle was professionally capable of doing the work required in Cherub, but there are other considerations relating to living in a children's home, and what might also be required in terms of Christian witness to the children, and any other responsibilities. Also, Besaniya Children's Home comes under the auspices of the Church of Uganda, although Africare has been solely responsible for all funding from the very start. This relationship wasn't always easy, and we had to work on it. It would have been easy at times to think of becoming totally independent but that could have presented a lot of difficulties. We always felt it was best to work closely with the national church, particularly as the time would come when much more responsibility would have to be taken locally. It isn't always easy for people from different denominations to fit into life in the Church of Uganda, and this was one of the issues we had to address with Danielle. Some concerns had also been raised by the diocese about having other denominations working at Besaniya, although I felt this was unfair. Very few of the people we sent to work at Besaniya, or who funded all the work, were Anglicans, yet we had always done our utmost to play a full and active role in the local church.

In drawing up the detailed job description for Danielle's consideration, we had some problems over the relationship with the Church of Uganda, and it seemed at that time that Danielle might not be the right person for the job. I wasn't happy about this, as I felt we were doing all we could to accede to the wishes of the diocese but that they weren't being as helpful as they might. This left us with a problem. If we couldn't have Danielle, what were our options? Florence had at times made use of a Ugandan physiotherapist, Paul Ochen, who seemed very capable. But Paul wasn't fully qualified, and there remained a question mark over his experience. We weren't sure if he was ready so soon to take over the running of Cherub, so we had to find someone. Again, a nurse or physiotherapist could have been suitable. A physio seemed ideal, but a nurse could have run the unit, with Paul dealing with physiotherapy.

Matters came to a head when Florence wanted to leave some months earlier than planned to get married. The pressure was on, and we had to do something. I was in Uganda around this time and had some difficult meetings with the diocese about the running of Besaniya and Cherub. I felt at the time that they were being unrealistically rigid in some of their requirements, as we had done all we could down the years to work in co operation. I saw this as a 'blip' and not indicative of our overall relationship with the church. Our work, particularly with ECM, was wide ranging and by now covered six dioceses, and we enjoyed excellent relationships. Denominational differences, for example, had never been an issue, we had always been able to work alongside each other as brothers.

The discussions we had were difficult and it seemed it could take some time to resolve anything. The need to find a replacement for Florence was becoming more pressing, so we felt we couldn't wait indefinitely. I once again contacted Danielle, explained the situation, and proposed a less detailed job description which left more to her own discretion. Danielle accepted this, and I hoped that the Church of Uganda would also go along with it for the sake of the work.

I was sorry to encounter these difficulties with the church, but perhaps it shouldn't have been surprising. The diocesan divisions mean a lot in Uganda but coming from outside, we saw things differently and took a much broader view. People in Mukono diocese were concerned with what happened in their own area, we were working across six dioceses. This then presented serious difficulties with handing over more control on a local basis. It was all a learning experience, and we were able to get through it. We were fortunate in having good friends high up in the Church of Uganda who can advise us with these difficulties. It wasn't just Danielle, this was a period of significant change at Besaniya involving other personnel, and changes in the management structure of Besaniya. This came at a time when there was also change in the church leadership, and we all had to get used to working together – we all depended on each other, so we had to develop a working relationship. This was a desperately stressful time for us. We had spent years developing Besaniya, and these differences could have placed it all in jeopardy – we simply had to find a way to continue to work together.

Danielle was able to make her arrangements quite quickly, and came to Uganda a very short time before Florence left. Some people would have preferred a longer overlap, but I'm not sure that's the best way. Of course, there were things Florence needed to show Danielle, but Florence had run Cherub her way, now it was time for Danielle to run it as she saw best. There was of course continuity with Harriett, and also with Paul still available on a part time basis. Janet McNickle from Northern Ireland had been there as a volunteer for nearly a year sharing the house with Florence, and assisting in Cherub much of the time. She stayed on, so was also able to help Danielle settle in. They were familiar with how everything was done, and could give Danielle guidance.

With modern communications, it was also very easy to contact Florence or ourselves if Danielle wanted to ask a question. Ease of communications – emails, mobile phones etc – can seem like a big advance, but it can be a double edged sword. There are times when we need to contact someone urgently, but at other times it may make it too easy for people to pass on problems instead of taking action or making decisions themselves. This wasn't the case with Danielle, she quickly got to grips with the work of Cherub and just got on with the job. There were others though who, in a period when we wanted more responsibility to be taken locally, kept contacting us for decisions on all kinds of matters. I think this problem grew gradually, it couldn't be blamed on any one person or event, but once we realised the problem we were able to deal with it, and changed a number of our procedures to effectively distance ourselves a little from 'day to day' running of the work.

Danielle's way of doing things was different from Florence's, but Cherub was none the worse for that. When Florence went there, she had to work with a completely new unit, and newly recruited workers. When Danielle arrived, the routine and procedures were pretty well established. While Florence had to develop the work, Danielle's role was one of consolidation, finding out exactly what others were capable of, and starting the process of giving them more responsibility. There was the usual worry of how a new worker would relate to everyone, not just in Cherub but in Besaniya, but Danielle at least had some previous experience in Uganda, and quickly settled in.

Once again, we had found the right person at the right time – but we're human, and always worried about what would happen if it didn't work out. With Danielle, as with Florence, we didn't have an alternative to fall back on. Danielle agreed to work with us for one year. We hoped at times that she'd agree to stay longer but she had other plans and it wasn't to be. So before long we were starting to think again about replacement staff. This time, was there any alternative to us sending someone out?

Danielle writes:

7th January 2003:
"It is amazing that it's already a month since I have been here. In the beginning, it seemed a bit challenging to adjust to everything. I thank the Lord for my previous experience but somehow the new people, new location, new responsibilities (such as driving the vehicle) proved to be a bit stressful at times. And I am very thankful for Janet, she has been a great help. In the two weeks that Harriett was away for Christmas holidays, Janet has been an assistant at Cherub. I think she has a talent for wound and foot care. To be honest, I haven't come across someone so eager to "get in there" for this type of work. She truly enjoys it in a way that I haven't seen before!

"I am slowly getting to know Sam and Mary, the Kizzas and their families. I have been getting to know Harriett and Janet more it seems, given the time I spend with them.

"Now for the work at Cherub, - I am truly enjoying it. It's been quite rewarding for me to see that some of my previous work at Katalemwa was remembered. There's something truly gratifying about being responsible for something. I'm still amazed at the gift that God has given me in trusting me with Cherub."

15th January 2003:

"I am now writing to you while looking at the most amazing sunset. I live and work on the west side of Besaniya Hill, near Kampala, Uganda. Before me is the most amazing view. I can see Lake Victoria in the distance and the sun bursting with orange as it sets into clouds all pink and purple.

"On a work level, I must admit that it has been challenging. As I only had four days with the previous physiotherapist who was here, it meant that I had to fend for myself. I consider it a blessing to have been so dependent on the Lord. There are currently 16 children in the rehab unit, with another 8 to come in the next few weeks. Then there are the children from the surrounding communities who come as out patients. At times I'm put in the role of physician as I decide which medication and dosage to give the children. Other times, I'm doing some nursing as I change dressings for wound care. But most often, I find myself in the more familiar role of physiotherapist as I assess and treat conditions that are primarily orthopaedic and neurological in nature."

23rd February 2003:

"Well, the work at Cherub has certainly kept me busy and challenged. Given the wonderful work that Florence has done, the word is out in some of the surrounding communities. Once a patient returns to their village, it isn't uncommon for a child from the same village to arrive as a new patient.

"I brought Saidi (former Cherub patient) to see Dr Fulvio (the orthopaedic surgeon who replaced Norgrove Penny). His tibia now needs to be lengthened but the prognosis is not good. Because the infection is so extensive and long term, it can still be with him for years. The other option is amputation; everything above his right tibia is healthy and infection free."

27th February 2003:

"Although you'd think putting 16 children together for an extended period of time can create a chaotic environment, I would say that it has been very much the opposite. Children with disabilities undergo a lot of discrimination and can experience a lot of rejection in their villages. I believe it stems from a lack of knowledge around disabilities. It's a common belief that a disability is a curse on the family. Hence, some children are kept hidden and even killed. I can't help but think that the children feel very much part of a community at Cherub. They feel accepted and have a sense of belonging."

2nd April 2003:

"I was invited to a nearby parish to assess the children in the community. When Harriett and I arrived there were 75 children waiting. Thirty five of them were booked into Cherub over the next few months, the others were helped on site or redirected to other health care professionals."

8th August 2003.

"I have gone on two more outreaches since last writing, one in a town called Nyanga, the other named Namiliiri. One of the children found through the outreaches is Lydia Nekesa. She is 6 years old and has cerebral palsy with severe spasticity in all limbs. Her family had never come across anyone who could help her so for all of her life she has been lying on her back. She stayed at Cherub for a few weeks. After one week of sitting in a seat she started gaining some head control. After two weeks, she was able to sit out of the chair with some assistance. She has now been discharged, but will be coming back. Her father said that prior to coming to Cherub he had lost hope and wasn't even feeding Lydia much any more. Everyone in the village was very surprised at the change in her."

From Danielle's last report prior to leaving Cherub in December 2003:

"The need for rehabilitative services is great here for children with disabilities. Most families don't have the finances that would allow their child to receive treatment. Even if they find the money for transport to certain facilities, they are often faced with bribes for medical practitioners to get the care the child deserves. Finances aside, a child with disabilities is faced with much stigma from their community and sometimes even their own family. The disability is seen as a curse and can lead to abandonment of the child.

"Peter is a 14 year old boy who came to Cherub crawling because of polio related problems; he had been crawling for most of his life. Following surgery to release his contractures, plaster work to complete the lengthening of the muscles, exercise and the fitting of braces and crutches, he left Cherub walking and able to meet people eye to eye.

"Akim is a 15 year old boy born with a condition called osteogenesis imperfecta / brittle bone disease, a condition in which bone density is greatly diminished hence the bowing and misshaped bones that can be easily fractured. Although he is 15 years of age, he is only about two feet tall. The condition brings a lot of pain and severe functional limitation (use of his hands only, not his arms, and lifting his head for short periods of time).

Through Cherub he received assistance in pain management, and a specialised wheelchair made at Katalemwa. He is now attending school

"Geoffrey is a 13 year old boy, one of the many children with club feet that have gone untreated. Following surgery and the use of plasters to fully reposition his feet, he left Cherub a happy teen with feet fitted in a new pair of shoes.

"If I was to describe the work in Cherub, I would say that it is primarily a 'mission of mercy' in that Cherub workers are exemplifying Christ in helping the poor and needy. It has been a blessing to not only share about Him through the meeting of the children's physical needs, but also through Bible teaching, prayer and worship which take place on a daily basis at Cherub.

"I can't tell you how crucial it was for me to follow the Lord's guidance to serve Him by helping children in a developing country. The work was incredibly satisfying. It meant the world to me to help children that are greatly in need through my physiotherapy skills.

"In the last year, 233 children have been assessed; we have admitted 62 children affected primarily by the following: cerebral palsy, club feet, osteomyelitis, post-injection paralysis, cleft lips, burn contractures, hip pathologies, birth deformities.

"Cherub has continued with the weekly cerebral palsy clinic. Two plastic surgery clinics have been conducted through the Katalemwa Cheshire Home. These clinics have addressed primarily conditions such as cleft lips, contractures as a result of burns or other trauma, and birth deformities.

"Kityo Robert is a 7 month old baby affected by a cleft lip and palate. He had difficulty feeding from his mother's breast before the operation. The care of these children is quite simple in that it is a matter of co-ordinating the visits for the surgical repair of the lip and palate. The post op care is minimal and the benefit to the child is very significant."

25.

THE NURSE

There were three options. Send a physiotherapist. Send a nurse. Or hand over to a local physiotherapist. Paul Ochen continued to do completely satisfactory part time work, but we still didn't feel the time was right to completely hand over. Sending another physiotherapist seemed the best choice, but I wasn't so sure. We were keen to start making more use of Paul, and perhaps broadening the community work, so I thought we should send a nurse. Either would have done though. For every problem, there's an 'ideal' solution, and there's the reality of what we have available. At this point, we had neither.

Some time before, we met a nurse from N Ireland, Denise Kane, who saw the work of Cherub while in Uganda with a work team. She was experienced, and had specialist training with children, but when we talked to her about Cherub she was quite clear that it wasn't the right place for her to be. It was also clear she wasn't going to change her mind – but I thought she was the ideal person for the job, so we had to try to convince her! Much later, when the need to find a replacement for Danielle was becoming more urgent, we once again asked Denise. I think we put pressure on her by making it clear we had no alternative! Thankfully, Denise accepted. This was a worry too however, because she had responded to our persuasion, and I didn't know how she would feel when she'd been there for a while. It's a big responsibility sending someone to work overseas, but a much bigger one when we try to convince them to do something they initially thought wasn't right for them.

I needn't have worried. Denise had only been there a short time when she wrote to thank us for persuading her to go, and saying that she believed she was now definitely in the right place. There were though some other issues to deal with. There had been a lot of debate about whether to send a nurse or physiotherapist. As well as a nurse being the only person available at the time, I still felt that a nurse manager was the right person. Of course a lot of the work was physiotherapy, but there was more to it than that, and we still had Paul available too. Now that the work had been effectively consolidated by Danielle, we could look to the future, and it fell to Denise to find exactly what our local staff were capable of, and also to what extent we could work out into the community. Florence had started this with various rural clinics, but Denise as an experienced nurse had the potential – and the desire – to develop it.

We were fortunate that, as with her predecessors, Denise quickly settled in and formed excellent relationships in Besaniya and Cherub. This meant a lot, as from the very start the work of Cherub would have been seriously undermined if people didn't get along on a personal level as well as having respect for each others capabilities. Where Florence developed the work and Danielle consolidated it, Denise had the gift of really getting the best out of everyone. We can now see, looking back, how at every stage of the work we had the right person and Cherub not only functioned very effectively from day one, but gained the confidence and admiration of all who came in contact with it.

By this time Harriett had gained a lot of experience. Although she started as a 'carer' or 'assistant', her willingness to learn, and to undertake whatever work was needed, meant she could now serve as assistant manager. Paul had also gained a lot more experience. Not only was his work of a high standard, but he cared deeply about the children, and had the confidence and respect of their parents. He still didn't have a proper job description but could be relied on to do much more than would normally be expected. Despite his lack of a professional qualification, he clearly had the potential to take more responsibility.

With all this in mind, we discussed with Denise the possibility of developing more work in the community. There was a big need for this, and Denise was very keen to get on with it. It also had the advantage of getting Denise out of Cherub more, leaving both Paul and Harriett to run clinics, make decisions etc. Everyone responded very well to this, and it was another step forward for Cherub.

Denise continued to build on the community work started by Florence. Sometimes this led to further referrals to Cherub, at other times particular needs were targeted such as dealing with refugees, or feeding programmes for children. The work of Cherub was soon widely known, and much more far reaching than we'd ever hoped. We could see clearly now that Denise had been the right person for the job and that she had brought Paul and Harriett to the stage where they were capable of running Cherub.

Although doing everything we could have asked of her in Cherub, it was evident that Denise's heart was very much in community work. We at one time hoped to be able to develop a separate base for community health work, but soon realised we were in danger of overreaching ourselves and also getting too far away from our original aims. Denise had agreed to serve for two years. Had we been able to develop a community health work, I think she would have stayed but her work in Cherub was done, and by late 2005 she was ready to leave. At least this time we already knew what came next and were able to work towards a handover to Paul and Harriett.

Denise writes:

29th January 2004:

"Abdul is a 12 year old boy who has become a Christian following exposure to the gospel in Cherub and attending a mission once discharged from Cherub. His father is dead and he lives with his mum and brother. When his mum heard that he had become a Christian she bit him, ripped his clothes and sent him from the house. The situation has got worse as she has approached the local council and accused Abdul of abusing her. He doesn't understand all that is going on and is homeless now. Please pray for this new young believer, it is a big test so soon after accepting Christ. Please pray for Sam, Harriett and I as we seek to sort out the situation and try to get him back home.

"Last week we attended an outreach clinic just outside Mukono, at Nakapinyi, which is home to about 200 Northern refugee women (mostly widows with the trouble in the north), and about the same number of children. We came across a child called Asaf with cerebral palsy. He looked tiny, but we discovered he was actually 6 years old. Very malnourished and dehydrated. The problem is twofold – neglect and poverty. We have admitted the boy and his mum so that we can feed and build up the boy and educate the mum in his care. When I asked if there were any more children like this I was told yes. I asked again about how many, I was told 10. Yet none of them was brought to the clinic. Obviously I need to find them.

"In this area there is a lot of HIV and Aids (children and adults). Please remember these widows and their children as they have very little materially to cater for their needs. Pray that in some way we will be able to help alleviate some of their suffering."

6th February 2004:

"I have been learning a lot in my short time at Cherub regarding the conditions and treatments necessary for the orthopaedic problems these kids have. I do feel that now is a good time for development of the work of Cherub, looking at the whole child and not just the disability, and for this time a nurse seems to be the person for the job. There are a lot of admin and nursing issues that need structure and organisation at Cherub, and there is generally a lot of need on our doorstep particularly in preventative medicine. I have been shocked and saddened by the number of children with cerebral palsy who were mismanaged by parents or quack doctors when their child had a fever. I have done a lot of networking and have met with directors from Mukono Health district. There is a lot to be done. The district has good intentions but nothing is happening on the ground. A familiar story.

"20 minutes outside Mukono we have people displaced from the North and also Congolese people who have fled from the conflict there. They have no money, many are HIV orphans and a majority of the parents are grandmothers, widows or single mothers. Asaf's mother is a widow with another child of 10 years. She has no means of support other than digging where she can get the work. Asaf's diet was sweet potato and tea. When they had money, he got sugar in his tea. When we discovered 6 year old Asaf, he weighed less than a 1 year old should. Every day he is improving, laughing, smiling and wanting more attention.

"I intend to go with Sister Mary to Kasenge village on Monday, where there are supposedly 10 children as bad as Asaf. In one village, Sr Mary and I have started a feeding programme for malnourished children, some with HIV. The need is great but we are working with local councillors and churches to assist them."

20th February 2004:

"The days are just flying in here, I can't believe that already we are nearly at the end of February. In Cherub, the work is going on well. We have a full house most nights, with children receiving post operative care and rehabilitation therapy. During the week we have two very busy outpatient days, Monday and Thursday. On a Tuesday I take kids in to see Dr Fulvio for a review or assessment for surgery. For anyone with a knowledge of orthopaedics I was amazed to find that here they remove orthofixes at the outpatient clinics! No anaesthetic or Calpol, the kids actually help to loosen the screws etc and off they come.

"We have been to three villages so far for outreach clinics and here we see kids with all sorts of maladies, chronic and acute. I really have to wonder at how some of these kids survive, especially neglected illnesses. I see kids with abdomens drum tense and distended and the carers casually tell you that they have been like this for years!

"There are many kids in the community with Downs Syndrome and I have yet to find a parent who has been told by any medical personnel that their child has a genetic disorder and what to expect for the future. I will try to get a lot of these families together so that they can support each other. I have never had to break news like this to people before and it is quite daunting.

"There is an obvious need for health education regarding preventable disease like cerebral palsy resulting from cerebral malaria which has been neglected or mismanaged. There is also an obvious need for spiritual care in these very badly affected areas, especially Nakapinyi. The little boy Asaf I mentioned previously is doing well and is now very responsive to his environment, laughing and smiling. He has a cataract which we are getting sorted out for him, and are also accessing a cerebral palsy chair before we send him home. I can't judge his mum too harshly as she has had a very difficult life. In fact during their time at Cherub she has lost the 'dead' look in her eyes, and is now laughing and enjoying the company and example of the other women here.

"There are real areas of spiritual need around us, and in Cherub we see kids from different religious backgrounds. We have daily opportunities to share the gospel with the kids and the carers through daily devotions, evening prayers and hopefully a good example on our part.

"It has come to my attention that there is a lot of witchcraft in the district of Mukono which has snuffed out other ministries and attempts to take ground for God. It has made me more aware of the battle that we are engaged in. Please pray first and foremost for the light of God's word to pierce the darkness here, I believe it is the key to any other work that we do here."

May 2004:

"David is 18 months old and weighed 4.5Kg when we found him at an outreach clinic. We admitted him to Cherub for treatment and a consultation with a paediatric consultant for some of his problems. He was put on oral antibiotics, multivitamins and high-energy porridge. At the end of his first week in Cherub he became ill very suddenly and we found that his mother hadn't reported his diarrhoea to anyone; in addition he had developed malaria, anaemia and pneumonia. In his malnourished state disease took advantage very quickly. The local hospitals couldn't assist as they had no blood to transfuse him. I had to drive like a maniac to Mengo Hospital in Kampala to get treatment for him. Despite being a better equipped hospital, they didn't have the necessary intravenous drip, and we had to visit eight different pharmacies before getting what we needed. David's mother has made no secret of the fact that she doesn't really care about David and wants a 'real' child, one who is not sickly or the result of an unwanted pregnancy. She is also waiting for the results of an HIV test.

"The outreach at Nakapinyi continues every Friday, with increasing numbers of families attending. There are more people arriving from the north of Uganda every month and the children have skin diseases etc on arrival as the journey down has been difficult. The increasing numbers have been quite overwhelming some weeks, and people's expectations are high. Sam Mutumba has also been required to act in response to medical emergencies in the area. He has also linked up with the lay reader and is doing a great work to encourage the church at Nakapinyi. The church is next to the school and there are no proper pit latrines, so Sam has mobilised the community to assist with building the toilets."

June 2004:

"David, the little boy who was malnourished and quite ill last month, has been discharged. He had gained weight and was eating well. His mum appeared thankful, and the family were pleased at the improvement in David, but I feel they could have done more to help long before David came to us.

"I spoke to Abdul's mum yesterday, apparently he is at school and generally doing well. However, a local minister informed me that his mum still restricts him from attending Christian worship.

"Thirteen year old Flavia had a flare up of her osteomyelitis and required further surgery last month. The surgical wound has cleared up, but she has pain in her ankle, affecting her ability to walk and making her miserable. As she has been with us for some time we decided to take her home for a few nights as she seemed depressed and homesick. Her stepfather refused to let us take her to the house, and told us to speak to her mother first. Flavia then confessed that the stepfather mistreated her and her younger brother. Because of the tension in the home Flavia and her brother now live with their grandmother. The stepfather has told them that if they ever come to the house again he will kill them. The mother told us she visits Flavia and her brother every day after work.

"We have had an immunisation clinic at Nakapinyi. This should have been the responsibility of another health centre, funded by the ministry of health. In reality, the money does not filter down to the grass roots level, therefore the clinics don't happen. If the clinics don't happen then we end up seeing children with illnesses like polio and TB."

15th October 2004:

"The Nakapinyi feeding programme continues with a positive change in the children, but we came across one girl called Christine. She is 8 years old but looks about 90, just skin and bones. We believe she is suffering from Aids. Her situation is a sad one. She is the sixth of eight children, the eighth just born this week. All have different fathers, but none seem to hang around. Her mother refused to send her to the feeding programme so the food was sent to the house, but they didn't give it to her. We went to the house and brought the girl out, the neighbours were astounded because they hadn't realised she was there.

"Christine was obviously uncomfortable and generally sore.· We treated her chest infection, gave some rehydration salts and pain relief. We counselled the mum and encouraged her to look after the girl, and said we would try to help them. That was two weeks ago. I am pleased to say there has been a slight improvement with the good diet and love being shown to her. The vomiting has settled and her chest is clear. She still needs a lot of care. Pray for a change in the mother's attitude, that she won't disregard her because of her illness but will instead love her children and change her lifestyle.

"Another family lost a little nine month old baby this week. The mum took the baby into a dangerous part of the forest to gather firewood. Apparently they are not meant to go there because of wild pigs. However the mother was desperate to get money so she went to gather firewood. The baby was set down on the ground while the mother collected the firewood but a wild pig came and attacked the child. Unfortunately they were not able to save the baby; the mother was hurt but should recover. Times are very hard for the people here as they will risk anything to earn a little money."

December 2004:

"Well it's December again and I have now been at Cherub for one year. The year has flown by, full of challenges, ups and downs, but praise God, He has been faithful in every circumstance. The large shops in Kampala are getting into the festive season but out in the villages life just continues with no deviation from the norm. There is no expectation of gifts or new clothes, no holiday break. However there will be a church service to celebrate the birth of Christ, and then if they are fortunate they may receive meat or rice instead of the usual maize and beans.

"At Nakapinyi the refugees will know some kindness and comfort this Christmas. Thanks to all your kind donations we are giving out more aid, including blankets and basic essentials. One family had one blanket between nine; now everyone in that home will have a blanket. There was a thanksgiving service at Nakapinyi for all that has been done in their school, village and church. There's health care for the kids, the school completed and extended by Fields of Life, and the church encouraged by the work of ECM through Sam and Mary Mutumba. The very poor have also received basic requirements through Africare's donors.

"This year in Cherub we have seen over 200 new patients. A monthly clinic at Kangalumira has been established in conjunction with Youth with a Mission where we assess, treat and advise kids with orthopaedic conditions and cerebral palsy. Recently we have begun to regularly visit some patients who cannot travel to Cherub because of their disability or social circumstances. It's been rewarding to see how this has encouraged and offered hope to families who felt forgotten and helpless."

March 2005:

"Kiggunda Fred is a seventeen year old boy who has been diagnosed since attending Cherub with muscular dystrophy. We met him at one of our outreach clinics 20 miles out from Mukono. Fred became a Christian in 2000, he felt touched when someone preached and made the decision for Christ. Before becoming a Christian Fred cursed his life and believed that God could not love him because of the way he looked. Fred's problem began when he was four, he developed weakness in his lower limbs and eventually was unable to walk. His family never sought treatment for him at any stage.

"Fred comes from a big family, his father produced 18 children, had three wives, not including the women he 'loved outside' as Fred put it. Fred was the youngest of three children of one of the wives but his mother left when he was six months old, he wouldn't even recognise her now. The stepmother did not treat him well and along with the father they believed it would be a waste of money to send him to school. They did eventually send him, but very late, then in P5 his father suddenly discontinued his education and sent him and two brothers to the village to live with the grandmother, who died 4 years ago.

"At school Fred was shown how to repair shoes and this is what he has been doing. However in the village people can little afford his services or take a long time to pay. In a day he can earn 700Ug Sh which is less than 30 pence. This has to buy food, soap, clothes etc.

"Fred hopes that when his treatment is finished he will walk and be able to take shoes around and sell them. He is enjoying his time at Cherub as he has the opportunity to eat different types of food that he hasn't had to strain for. He says a big thank you to all the people who have been involved in his treatment and well being.

"We are in the process of using plaster of Paris to stretch and straighten Fred's legs. He will probably need callipers to support his legs, and the disease is progressive. Please keep Fred in your prayers, for his healing, and also that he might realise his dream to work and be fully self sufficient."

10th June 2005:

"Bubumba John is a cheeky wee 7 year old who was successfully treated at Cherub for bilateral club feet. At a recent outreach clinic he attended for follow up with his mum. We found out that when he went home, on the Sunday he told his mum in no uncertain terms that he was saved and they were going to church – so his mum has started taking him.

"Bosco, 15, was successfully treated for post polio paralysis. He had contractures of the knees and ankles because of the disease. He went home last week on callipers and crutches where before he had been crawling and looking up from the ground. The reception we received from the family and community was overwhelming and God was praised for the work done on his legs. They sent us away with corn, pineapples, matooke, chickens, avocado etc. It was so much from a very poor community, it was wonderful.

"Rose Nansubya is 18 years old and recently had a tumour removed from her knee. The biopsy has shown it to be an osteosarcoma, therefore she will need further help. We hope to take her to an oncology clinic next week to rule out spread and organise further management of the disease."

3rd November 2005:

"I am writing in the midst of packing up house. I can't believe how quickly the last two years have gone. I'm looking forward to going home, but don't think the change will truly hit me until I am home for a while and reality has set back in. My successor is Joyce Kayaga, a local nurse who will take over the leadership and management of Cherub with the help of Paul and Harriett. It can be so overwhelming to step into this role as it is specialised in comparison to general nursing. Please remember Joyce as she takes over, pray that God will strengthen her, grant her wisdom and discernment and bind all three into a strong team.

"I don't know how to thank everyone for all the support I have had during these last two years. To all who have given to the work of Africare thank you again, a little goes a long way out here. Many have given for specific things which has been wonderful, but thank you to all the people who have also given for the ongoing work which is so important."

26.

PAUL

When Denise replaced Danielle in Cherub, it became necessary for Paul to deal with all the physiotherapy. He was coming in for three days each week, but we would have liked him to do more, or to come to work for us full time. We knew this would be a big step for him as there was some security, including pension rights, with his government work and Cherub was still very new. Continuing to work part time meant he had to put in very long hours to deal with the work, but he never complained. We did feel though that there was more to his wish to only work part time for us, and to keep up his other work, and we eventually understood what he was concerned about.

From the start, Paul was used to working in Cherub as an assistant physiotherapist, first with Florence, then with Danielle. They were very experienced and professionally qualified, he wasn't. Now, with Denise there, he was still expecting us to send out another physiotherapist so that he would still be an assistant. We hadn't said anything about this to him, but I think he heard from others that a replacement physio was being sought. By now we were confident enough of Paul's skills, and of Denise's ability to manage Cherub, that we had no intention of sending a physiotherapist out. I wrote to Paul explaining this, and saying that as far as we were concerned he was now the Cherub physiotherapist. We wanted him to know that he was central to the future of Cherub. Paul agreed to work one more day each week, and the work settled into a new routine – as far as anything there could be called routine – with Denise developing more community work.

When I next visited Cherub I could see for myself how effective the work now was. The community work had a big impact in a number of areas, and more children than ever were being treated in Cherub. Harriett was still a 'carer' in that she lived in the unit, to be available if any problems arose. She was also increasingly helping with administration and had learnt a lot from assisting with medical procedures. She was now able to carry out a range of work unassisted. Where previously the treatment room was used to deal with one child at a time, it was now possible to deal with three simultaneously. When I went there, I saw Paul carrying out a plaster change on one child, Harriett changing dressings on another, while Denise worked on a third child's external fixator. With a work like Cherub, with a small number of staff, it's vital that people are flexible and prepared to help where needed. Harriett was now much more than just an assistant, and had become a key member of staff. Some work was also delegated to long term patients, one of whom I saw serving as a 'ward orderly', dealing with practical arrangements and when I was there, making preparations for a new admission. Despite the sometimes chaotic appearance of such a crowded and busy unit, there was an underlying organisation and efficiency that spoke volumes about how it was being run.

Paul was also doing much more than could reasonably be expected of him. He would never leave a job unfinished, and was prepared to work long hours to complete everything before going home – not just dealing with the last patient, but leaving everything prepared for the next day. For Paul and Harriett we could see that Cherub was much more than just a job, and they were finding fulfilment through their work there.

In an ideal world Cherub might have had more staff or better facilities. Also, we were responsible for running the unit without ourselves having any medical experience. Because of this there were times when we were glad of an independent view of what we were doing. There are a lot of visitors to Besaniya so quite a few people have seen the work and spoken to us afterwards. While generally impressed, too many people kept suggesting we should do more, without thinking about how we could possibly do it. This is one of the problems of a 'successful' work, the demands just keep on increasing. Another problem with a work which looks good is that people assume it's well funded, and instead help something which looks a shambles, and they think is more in need of help. This ignores the fact that it may be a shambles because of poor administration or corruption. Our work has always functioned on a tight budget, and we continue to need all the help we can get – it's a tribute to our workers that it may look as if it's not in need of help!

Thankfully though, there were those who were prepared to help support what we were doing. We didn't mind being given advice, but it had to be realistic, taking into account our situation and resources. But however well intentioned these comments or advice, it wasn't the same as an expert assessment. We didn't want to 'spy' on our workers, they had to know we had confidence in them and of course we received regular reports from Cherub. What we needed was an evaluation which would be shared with all of them and could be a help to us in developing the work. Of course professionals like Florence, Danielle, Denise and Paul were constantly evaluating their own work and trying to improve it, but we wanted an overview.

On two occasions Agnes Magowan, a nurse practitioner, was able to do this for us. She travelled out to Uganda with her husband Raymond of Evangelical Ministries when he ran courses for us. Agnes then stayed at Besaniya and was able to see all the work of Cherub. She did this for the first time when Danielle was there. The work had been up and running for over two years so it was a good time to try to evaluate it all. Agnes was also able to give some instruction to Harriett on dressings, which was much appreciated. Agnes' comments were very worthwhile, she wasn't being unrealistic and asking us to do more but was looking for ways in which what we were already doing could be improved. I didn't involve myself too much in this although I was certainly very interested in Agnes' views. Instead, Agnes tried to show them in Cherub where there were any weaknesses, and where improvements might be made. In this way the staff could see that this was done for their benefit, rather than us seeking to find fault.

About a year later Agnes was able to visit again. She was very enthusiastic about the work and when I spoke to her afterwards she didn't raise anything she thought we should change. It was obvious that everyone concerned was doing their utmost to ensure all the work was carried out to a high standard, and there was certainly no sign of complacency. There was a recognition by everyone concerned of the consequences of working with sick children if everything wasn't done properly. Make no mistake, some of these children were very sick and we shouldn't underestimate the risks of working with them, or the level of care they required.

Paul writes:

1st July 2004:

"I love so much being part of Cherub, and being able to use my professional skills. I've had lots of disappointments in the past, and I went to Cherub reluctantly, but Denise was wonderful and has helped in bringing out my gift of healing which had been suppressed in my previous work.

"Because of her, I've been to Kasese, on the border with Congo, where we had a wonderful welcome from the family of a Cherub patient. He had complicated deformities of his lower limbs and had not walked for many years. He had been taken to many hospitals and the answer he always got, from Ugandan and expatriate doctors, was that nothing much could be done. However, to their surprise, we made him walk in Cherub. When we visited his home, they had a party for us with some people coming from Congo to see the people who had made the boy walk. There was also a thanksgiving service with prayers for all the work of Cherub, and their partners and donors. They brought lots of disabled children and wanted us to work on them immediately!

"I am pleased with what I have been able to do, but I give the credit to Denise. It's because of her humbleness, respect, and wonderful way of managing people that it's possible for me to do the work I do, and now we have miracles happening."

27.

THE 'CHERUB' CHILD

It's difficult for us to imagine what it is like for a child in Cherub, but it's worth considering the difference it can make for them and for their family. They are all individuals, and every case is different, but they will probably have a number of things in common. Whatever difficulty they have with their disability in terms of mobility, they may also have been rejected. This may mean they have a very poor relationship with their family and feel like rejects. They may never have been able to go to school, and in many cases may never have had the company of other children. For some, they will have been completely hidden away so that no one sees them. They therefore have very little idea of what the 'outside' world is like. There is nothing to look forward to. They can't engage in any of the activities 'normal' children enjoy. They have no stimulus. In fact they feel they aren't 'normal' at all, and have grown used to their status.

For others, the disability may have come later, after they have led a fuller life – and then it suddenly comes to an end – an accident, polio, post injection paralysis, burns contractures etc.

Of course there are many Ugandan parents who care deeply for their children regardless of disability, and there are disabled children who lead active lives despite their problems, but for many, it's hard to imagine what it is like for the parents. They have a disabled child. They may blame themselves; it's a curse; it's because of something they have done. They may not want the child; it's a burden; it's a stigma on the whole family; it has no future, won't be able to provide for itself; what are they going to do as it grows older? There may be pressures from 'traditional' doctors or even witch doctors to do something extreme – kill them, abandon them (thankfully rarer now, but it still happens) or spend money on 'cures' which achieve nothing or make things worse.

Such children may be brought to Cherub by their parents – this increasingly happens now that the work is becoming more widely known. Particularly in the early days though, they had to be sought out, sometimes following rumours.

So, by whatever means, the child is brought to the notice of Cherub and assessed. They are suddenly taken away from everything they have known – which may have been a very small 'world'. They are surrounded by strange faces, people whose language they may not understand poking and examining them, and then they are put in a vehicle and taken to Mengo Hospital for surgery. The journey alone may be terrifying for them – they are going into the unknown. Before they realise what is happening or are able to take in another set of surroundings, they go under anaesthetic and have surgery. When they waken, they have no idea where they are, they are again surrounded by strange people. For some, their parents will be with them, for others there is no one they recognise. They are probably in a lot of pain, and will have a plaster cast on which restricts their movement – they have no idea what it is or why it's there.

Then, just as they are trying to take it all in and grasp what they've been told about what has been done to them, they are taken from the recovery ward, loaded into a vehicle, perhaps with a number of others, and taken to Cherub. Their parents may or may not visit them; unless they are very young, no one they know will be staying with them. It's only a day or two since they underwent surgery, and suddenly there's another complete change of surroundings, it is all happening much too fast for them to understand or adjust. There is also the concern about what the plaster is, and what is going on inside it.

Yet we now see how resilient children can be. After a day and a night of feeling thoroughly miserable, in pain, terrified, they waken in a room full of other children and the change in them has to be seen to be believed. Children who may never had had contact with other children suddenly find themselves engaged in lots of activities with others in the same situation and it's a transformation. They make the adjustment so quickly, and their new situation becomes 'normal'. One of the remarkable things about Cherub is to see how joyful a place it is.

It is rarely quiet in Cherub and despite all the efforts of the staff it can be chaotic too. Up to 20 children of all ages, most quite young, many of whom haven't had the company of other children before; they can really make up for lost time. They very quickly learn how to play together, and they don't let their plaster or supports get in the way, they can be very active almost from day one. In the mornings, when they are all cleaned, dressed and organised (which takes some doing) they have breakfast – like all meals, it's taken in the dining hall with the Besaniya children, but it's probably the least 'social' meal of the day. Not everyone gets there on time, it's rushed as Besaniya children leave to go to school. When the Besaniya children have left, the Cherub children go to the classroom. There, they will sing choruses and hear a Bible story. A number of people at the home take turns to lead this. Usually the rest of the morning is taken up with lessons. We have a teacher for Cherub, and others may assist. For some children it may be the first time they have attended school; for others we try to make up for all the time they are missing from school. Throughout the day, treatment continues – a constant round of examinations, plaster changes, dressings etc. Some of the older children may assist as 'orderlies'. Soon it's lunch time – this is a fairly quiet meal, as most of the Besaniya children will be at school.

After lunch, there's a period of recreation – which looks positively dangerous. There's a lot of energy to burn off with various games and activities – again, plaster and appliances don't seem to inhibit them, and wheelchairs can attain remarkable speeds. There may be football, table tennis, badminton, while others are in the playground, on the swings and roundabout etc. The first play equipment at Besaniya was a tyre hanging on a rope from a tree to form a swing. I have seen up to five children swinging on this, with plasters sticking out in all directions. Then, with the help of a work team, a proper playground was constructed (and eventually replicated at Salaama for the blind children). By mid afternoon everyone is completely exhausted and they go back into Cherub for a sleep – this is the only time of the day Cherub is quiet.

Later, some 'quieter' activities are engaged in – playing with Lego in Cherub, perhaps board games, or reading in the library. The evening meal is the biggest of the day, both in terms of the quantity of food eaten, and the numbers present. I have counted up to 65 people in the dining room in the evening, with Besaniya and Cherub children, staff, and some parents. It's a more leisurely meal than others, finishing with choruses, prayers, perhaps a story or drama. Sometimes a video will then be shown, or the children have some time to themselves before bedtime.

It's a very full day for them, and their time in Cherub can be very enjoyable, certainly very different from anything they have previously experienced. However we need to keep in mind the environment they will be going back to, and we try to work with the parents and sometimes the community. We want the parents to recognise the child's value, and it is wonderful to see their attitude change as they realise the child isn't cursed, the disability wasn't their fault, and there is something they can do to help.

The stay in Cherub can be a long one for many of the children; we can't let them return home as they would probably never come back for outpatient treatment, or their plaster could be destroyed within a day. They are with us for long enough for us to see real change take place, not just for their physical condition but their spiritual and emotional development too. Usually we are happy to see them return home, but there are cases where their home circumstances cause us concern and we follow up with home visits to try to avoid problems and see them settled in an environment where their development can continue.

Whatever pain they suffered is usually short lived, so children can really enjoy their time in Cherub, but we have to be extremely careful with them, and with their parents, lest we create unrealistic expectations. We don't want them to experience conditions which won't be sustainable when they return home; for this reason, most play or education is based on being with other children, or using very basic equipment – we don't want them getting used to things they won't have outside of Cherub. We have a lot of visitors and volunteers passing through Besaniya, and well intentioned but misplaced generosity can be a problem too. We try to meet all the children's needs – but there are other things which aren't necessary, like new clothes or toys, which people sometimes try to provide for them. This can very quickly create the expectation that they will continue to receive help from us. We want to deal with their problems, rehabilitate them, and move on to deal with more cases, not get tied into more and more long term commitments. We don't want to give disproportionate help to some when there are others in such need. We constantly have to keep in mind Ugandan culture, traditions, values etc, and not make it more difficult for someone to return to 'normal' life at home. This has certainly been a problem at Besaniya, high expectations created and people expecting to keep on receiving help long after they should be fending for themselves.

This problem can be made worse by having expatriate workers. We expect expats to bring skills; often others expect them to bring other benefits too, and it is a difficult balance. Particularly with community work, it is better not to have it associated with expat workers, and we certainly try to avoid having expats give out any kind of direct help in the community – we try to use existing community structures for this. We can treat a Cherub child at very low cost; we can build a primary school, or do other community work, in a very cost effective way. However sponsoring one child, although it may start out cheaply, can become a very expensive exercise which it is difficult to conclude satisfactorily. It is all too easy to 'condition' a child, in effect make them a beggar. Unfortunately, many children in Uganda are steered towards expensive higher education or training, which may be totally inappropriate and simply a means of someone making money from them. We have had a lot of difficulty in the past convincing children to do appropriate skills training instead of wanting to do something we feel is a waste of time and money, and possibly beyond their capabilities. There are skills which are in great demand in Uganda, but they are not usually the ones the children want to train in.

We have been working there long enough now to see most of the problems, but also to see successes. We have seen children who find it very hard to break their dependency on Besaniya - it will always be their 'family', but we want them to be independent. But we have seen others really put their training to use and go on to do well. We are hoping it will be the same for Cherub. Many of the children we deal with would have had no hope for the future; they were destined always to be outcasts or rejects but having dealt with their physical needs, and hopefully having also dealt with the attitude of their parents and community to them, their full potential can be realised. This is something we will be looking at closely in the future.

One Cherub club foot patient was known by his whole village to be disabled, and no one imagined that would ever change. When he returned home walking normally and wearing shoes, people wanted to see his foot. The child saw an opportunity in this; anyone wanting to see had to pay for him to remove his shoe!

28.

THE DOCTOR

More recently, we had another opportunity for a professional assessment of the work. This was timely, as we near the handover to Ugandan staff. We want to be able to provide them with adequate back up, and address any remaining concerns about how the unit is run.

Dr Ian Ross from Florida was able to visit Cherub with John Cross, whose enthusiasm for the work remains undiminished, and who continues to help support it through the 'Upper Room' charity. While Agnes previously looked at our work form a broader medical perspective, Ian is a very experienced lecturer in physiotherapy and we welcomed the opportunity for an expert view. Following his visit Ian prepared a detailed report and recommendations. While he highlighted a number of weaknesses which we are now anxious to address, we were very encouraged by the overall tone of his report, which was a very supportive endorsement of our work. This is very encouraging and we believe that any criticisms he mentioned can be dealt with, and will improve the service we provide. Overall, his report is of considerable value as we prepare for the future. His positive comments will be welcomed by our staff; the weaknesses identified will enable us to take action now, and hopefully avoid more serious problems in the future. Any criticism is constructive, with the proposed solutions detailed, which is a big help.

Ian is experienced in Africa but the report in general, as we would have wished, looks at the care provided from the children's perspective, rather than from the limitations or difficulties of working in Uganda. We try to avoid settling for lesser standards just because of the location we work in or any associated problems. I know there are times in Africa when we simply can't do things the way we might like, but too often I hear 'Africa' used as an excuse for other failings or, which really upsets me, comments such as 'it's good enough', or 'it's better than they would have had otherwise.' If we are to build a relationship of trust with the people we work with, we must be seen to do our very best in their interest, rather than compromise. They do of course understand all the constraints of limited resources, manpower, specific local problems – but they will also understand very quickly if we try to give them 'second best.' All our work is intended as a Christian witness, so there is no excuse whatever for taking the 'easy' way, or for a lack of commitment. Also, of course, when dealing with the medical needs of children, any failings could have extremely serious consequences.

Ian's was a lengthy report and I'll just mention some of his observations, which I hope will give a fuller picture of the work as we prepare for the future.

"I had the opportunity to attend and participate in the Cherub rounds and outpatient clinic. My purposes for accompanying John on this trip were to see first hand the work done on behalf of the Upper Room, and to observe and make recommendations from the perspective of a physical therapist for Cherub as it is undergoing a transition to Ugandan staff. This very brief opportunity to see Cherub in action and to observe Paul, Harriett and Denise at work is the basis for the following observations and recommendations.

"Cherub is a 20 bed post surgery unit that primarily provides initial care to children who have undergone various surgical procedures, or are receiving serial-casting interventions. Cherub was initially set up in conjunction with the Uganda Orthopaedic Project as a site where post-operative care could be supervised and managed. Most of the care provided at Cherub involves some aspect of plaster or fibreglass casting. The unit is located in the grounds of the Besaniya Children's Home in Mukono, Uganda. Besaniya has been in operation for about 20 years, and Cherub started about 5 years ago.

"The physical plant at Cherub includes a large open plan dormitory room, a smaller semi-private dormitory room useful for patient isolation, indoor toilets and separate outdoor latrines and washing facilities. Patients share the dining, common room and classroom facilities of the adjoining Besaniya building. There is a table tennis table on the connecting verandah and a playground equipped with swings, a see-saw and roundabout in front of the building.

"Treatment facilities at Cherub consist of a simple treatment room equipped with two high-low plinths, cast cutting equipment, casting material, a desk, file cabinets, and bookshelf. Other equipment in the treatment room includes an autoclave, basic medicine, dressings, and other materials used for dressing changes. Running water for hand washing is available in the treatment room, as is an X ray viewing box mounted on the wall above the desk.

"Rounds are conducted at the bedside. The beds are set at a height appropriate for the children who sleep there, but as treatment or evaluation tables they are less than adequate. Outpatient clinics, dressing changes, cast fabrication and cast changes, and other interventions are performed in the treatment room. Patient consultation occurs in the treatment room with the patients and their parents seated on a bench beside the desk.

"Medical diagnoses of children cared for at Cherub have included: cerebral malaria (locally termed cerebral palsy), osteomalaria secondary to tuberculosis, and congenital equinas (club foot). Other care has been provided to children who have had limb lengthening surgery utilising the Lizarof procedure, limb contracture correction secondary to accidental burns and polio, injection paralysis requiring posterior tibialis tendon transfer, and fractures.

"Most care provided at Cherub involves intervention at the impairment level. This care treats problems of tissue structure and function. It includes wound care, dressing changes, cast care, and cast removal and fabrication.

"Interventions provided by the rehabilitation staff generally consists of care done to the patients. The children are however very active on the grounds and do not allow functional limitations to inhibit their level of activity. In this way they are, by necessity, very involved in their own care.

"Denise Kane appears to have quite a broad latitude to make treatment decisions, including dispensing medicine and referral to other practitioners. She has recently obtained use of the X ray facilities at Katalemwa, and through this relationship receives consultations from the physicians who staff the clinics there.

"Paul Ochen and Harriett appear to be equipped to provide the level of care currently available at Cherub. Both have been taught largely on the job, or have been self-taught. Paul has received some formal training during a previous employment situation, and has applied that training, as well as his own learning, at Cherub. Paul and Harriett each probably need some form of authentication or certification to ensure they continue to provide appropriate care, and have a source from which to modify the care they provide as the patient-mix changes."

Ian's observations on training and qualifications are something we were already aware of. For Cherub's registration with the Ministry of Health, there must be a qualified professional there. Up to now that has been the physiotherapist or nurse manager. Now that we are handing over, we are employing a qualified Ugandan nurse. Training in community based rehabilitation has been arranged for Harriett, and we will continue to look at possibilities for Paul. It's not appropriate to send him away for training. He is already very capable in what he is doing, and there is no point going to a lot of expense to have him train for procedures, treatments or equipment which aren't appropriate to his work at Cherub. It is our hope however that as medical training is introduced at the nearby Uganda Christian University, there may be other possibilities in future to enhance Paul's skills. Ian made some specific recommendations about this which we will look at carefully.

Ian then comes to conclusions, including the following extracts:

"Cherub is a fantastic operation. It provides needed care by local people in an environment that is well placed in the fabric of the local area. My impression is that Africare is effectively bridging the humanitarian – evangelism divide, and getting out of the way while Ugandans operate the projects. I saw Cherub as the hands and feet that are bringing good news to the people of Uganda. Cherub is a vehicle of evangelization. As such it serves a purpose far greater than simple rehabilitation. I do have some concerns about the quality and level of rehabilitation care being provided, and suspect that, with minimal input, the functional outcome to the children could be improved.

"Africare is spread across a wide range of interconnected projects. To expand the reach of Cherub into functional rehabilitation and assisting the children with the challenges they will face in their societal role may be appropriate. But, I do think that the idea of an offshoot into a rehabilitation curriculum may be too far removed from the central purpose of Africare. Nevertheless I offer it as a 'big picture' dream for a future project that could continue the process of returning Uganda to Ugandans. It would be a pleasure to assist Paul, Harriett, Cherub, Besaniya, Africare and the Upper Room in the future development of the rehabilitation side of things."

Ian's report is both encouraging and thought provoking, and we are grateful for the effort he put into it. It now falls to us to act on what he has said, as Cherub moves to the next phase of its work.

29.
VOLUNTEERS

The story of Cherub wouldn't be complete without some mention of those who have gone out to help for varying periods of time, whether individually or as part of a team. From the very start of the work at Besaniya, we have depended heavily on voluntary help and have had a large number of people of all ages and skills go out over the years to do whatever they could. We have been very glad of their efforts, and a lot of work has been done which we couldn't have managed otherwise.

Often, an individual could be placed to help in whatever way they could with ongoing work – perhaps giving practical help with buildings or maintenance, or helping with teaching. Some, with particular skills, have been able to use their time there to train others. We have also been very grateful to those who have been flexible and willing to fill any gaps, even though it was not what they expected or were prepared for. With the additional work of Cherub, Besaniya can be a busy place, and there are often occasions when staff are fully stretched and a volunteer is of value.

Then there are those who go as part of a team. This is often planned so that a larger project such as a building can be undertaken – and it can be very demanding. Few find it easy – everything is different, there's the culture, climate and food to adjust to as well as working very hard. Of course it doesn't make much sense to send out volunteers to do work which locals should be doing for themselves, but particularly in the early days of the work, following the years of suffering, there was a lack of motivation and often the work done by volunteers would encourage others to get started. There were times when a work team could give a lot of encouragement – it was always important that they worked alongside locals rather than simply going in and doing the job for them.

In more recent years, as the work has grown, there has been more emphasis on work teams and a number have been organised with Evangelical Ministries. Most of our bigger practical projects there have involved work teams who have not only provided skills but have helped raise money for the necessary materials. We are thankful that very few problems have arisen, particularly when we stop to think of all that could have gone wrong, sending so many people to sometimes remote locations, and a situation that was often entirely new to them. Much of what people saw could come as a shock to them but they rose to the challenge. Not only have they completed a lot of valuable work, but many were touched by what they saw and have remained involved. For many, even very experienced and well travelled people, what they experienced was life changing. Although they might have seen a lot in the past, what made the difference was that we tried to ensure they got to know people on a personal level and could come to understand them better. This was very important to Christians; they might have previously talked about their 'brothers in Christ' but it had remained a concept – now it became a reality. It was wonderful to see, on so many occasions, how someone started their work in Uganda thinking how different everything was, but came away realising how much they had in common.

A lot of work has to go into preparing teams to go out. It's not easy to adjust to seeing such deprivation and need. The problem is how to help, apart from completing the work they have gone out to do. Unfortunately, alongside the real and genuine needs there are people 'on the make' who can tell a very convincing story, and we always do our best to ensure that for anyone who wants to help, whatever they subsequently do will serve it's intended purpose. It can be all too easy for well intentioned, but ill advised, help to simply make people beggars. Many have remained involved with our work, and continue to provide financial support. Quite a few have also gone back, perhaps staying for longer – their initial experience has enabled them to prepare to help with some need they have identified. While many may never return, few will ever forget the experience. First impressions on going to Uganda can be very negative – they see poverty, suffering, need which can be almost overwhelming. However by the time they leave most people have a much more positive view. As well as seeing great need they will also have seen how much is being done, and what can still be done if enough people help. We particularly want them to see the efforts being made by many

Ugandans to bring about change.

It can be hard to imagine what one person could usefully do going out to a completely alien situation for perhaps just a few weeks. And I certainly don't want to compare the efforts of a short term volunteer with the commitment of those who undergo lengthy training and go on to give many years of service. It takes a very long time to truly understand another culture and its problems and be able to help effectively. But there is a need for all kinds of help, and provided the short term volunteer is prepared to place themselves under authority and do what they are told, a lot can be achieved. One person mightn't be able to do much, but a properly organised skilled team, for whom adequate preparations are made, can do a great deal in a very short time.

I can't mention here all that has been done by volunteers, but some of the projects are notable. The biggest building at Besaniya, the dining hall/classroom/office etc, was built by a work team. They found it very demanding, but they left a valuable work behind. We have also helped with work teams for Mengo Hospital and other medical projects. Work teams and individual volunteers have helped with ongoing work on various building projects at Besaniya, Salaama (with the blind children), Nakapinyi (with refugees) and on the islands. The school on Jana was put up by a work team – far from the ideal location to send a team to, but they rose to the challenge. The new Cherub wash block was also completed by a team.

It is very important that people go out for the right reasons. It's going to be tough for them both physically and emotionally and they have to be prepared adequately. We also need to be careful about their expectations, we don't want them to be disappointed because a building for example couldn't be completed in the time they were there. They become part of a chain, they use their skills for the time they are out, then someone else completes the work. Whatever 'work' they leave behind they need to understand the encouragement they can give just by being there to stand alongside people and try to identify with them.

Whatever we do to prepare people, they are still going to get a shock when they get there. We have them meet with people who have been out before, look at work done by previous teams, see films, get lots of background information. By the time they go, they will know quite a lot about Uganda, the people, the projects – but it still can't prepare them for the moment when they get off the plane and see it for themselves. Instead of seeing pictures or hearing stories, all their senses are assailed simultaneously by the sights, sounds and smells of Africa. Even at Besaniya there is never silence – everything from children by day to the sound of the insects at night, the birds and other wildlife early in the mornings, to the spectacle of an African thunderstorm. Many things take them by surprise but it's a wonderful experience. They will have fears about going there, but these usually fade into insignificance when they experience the reality, the problems usually occur when they get back home.

Particularly for those going out for a short time, it's a very intense experience with one new sensation coming on top of another. There is no let up, right through to boarding the plane home. But when they step off the plane at home, the reality hits them. There will be the usual problems of relating our indulgent society and culture to what they have just seen, there is just so much to absorb, much of which they hadn't really time to think about when they were there. There will be many memories too of people they met; real concerns for them, and a desire to help. Perhaps a lasting impression of how much some people are doing so unselfishly in the face of adversity. But there is also a sense of 'did it really happen', and I know quite a few people have real trouble adjusting when they return. When friends and family ask 'what was it like', how can they start to describe what they really felt and experienced? We always try to warn people that their biggest problem won't be adjusting to Africa, but adjusting to 'normal' life when they get back.

This can be a costly exercise too, and a number of people have asked whether it would be better simply to donate the cost of their fare. We have thought about this, but I think our experience has shown that it has been much better to go there; give whatever help is possible, but come back having learnt something that will always be of benefit, and may enable them to be of much more help in the future. As well as those who have remained linked to our work, we have seen many people go on to help with other projects, perhaps in other countries, because of their initial experience with the work in Uganda. As well as the growth we have seen with our own work over the years, we have seen a lot of other work established which is linked to us in some way.

We hope to continue sending work teams in the future; a number of people who were previously out on teams now give a lot of help in recruiting and preparing groups to go out, and we are identifying a number of projects where they could be used. The trend is towards much smaller teams of skilled people who may be able to help in more remote locations, and could give a lot of encouragement.

30.

JANA

With Cherub established, we wanted to cast the net as widely as possible, and one way we saw of doing this was to involve ECM workers. Evangelical Christian Ministries, from very small beginnings, now covered a very large area and we had a widespread network of associate workers. Under the direction of Patrick Wakkonyi and Sam Mutumba, suitable candidates had been identified and joined ECM as associates, taking on a leadership role in their own area. These associates would be responsible for organising missions and training programmes, and the work was in great demand from the Church of Uganda.

The work of ECM was run from an office beside the bishop's house at Namirembe, where Patrick met regularly with a group of 'senior' associates – each a co-ordinator for their own diocese. Together they discussed the strategy for the work. We also had a house in Kampala, occupied by Patrick and his family, which served as a base for residential training courses. We believed that what distinguished ECM from the many other evangelical agencies was our very close relationship with the Church of Uganda and the importance we placed on the follow up training of new converts. A range of training programmes were offered for this purpose. We also concentrated a lot of effort on the ongoing training of our associates, the aim being to have a core of well trained workers who were properly equipped to lead and to train others. This policy had been very successful, and ECM continued to grow. It was logical to make these people aware of the work of Cherub so that they might be able to pass on information about suitable cases in their own areas. Sometimes, a disabled child would be brought to us, particularly as news of the work spread. In other cases, we had to go and find them sometimes following rumours about a disabled or injured child.

Many of the ECM associates have now been informed of the work of Cherub; they are working in many areas, and coming in contact with people who because of distance or poverty would rarely seek medical attention. Some of the most deprived areas are on the islands in Lake Victoria, and much of the ECM effort has been directed there in recent years.

Most of the indigenous people left the islands years ago; the people there now are a mixture, having gone out for various reasons, often to escape something. They live by fishing, and on the more remote islands it's a tough existence with a very poor quality of life. We were surprised to find so little sense of community, most were living as individuals around the edge of the islands. We were also surprised at the accommodation, little attempt had been made at building suitable houses, instead most lived in shacks. On the mainland, even the poorest put some effort into building mud huts. It seemed that a lot of the people there were unwilling to admit that this was home. They imagined that they would make enough money from fishing to be able to move back to the mainland, so seemed unwilling to put the effort into building more permanent homes. Sometimes too there could be issues over land ownership, forcing them to put up only temporary structures. There is also a very high rate of HIV there, with a large percentage of the adults infected. Our fear is of the children following the same path, there is almost an inevitability about it unless something is done to improve the quality of life and change attitudes.

The first island ECM worked on was Jana, about 25 miles out in the lake with a population of around 1000. There had at one time been a church and a school, but I've no idea when these last functioned. Little remained of them. The ECM associates are highly motivated, and willingly went there to participate in missions. It's a difficult journey, the 'public hire' boats operating on the lake are crowded, uncomfortable, and often dangerously overloaded. They are also very slow, so it's a lengthy journey during which weather conditions can change dramatically.

The first mission on Jana bore fruit, with a number of dramatic conversions which proved to be a big influence on others. One woman who practised witchcraft and organised sacrifices on the islands became a convert, and subsequently went through several of the ECM training courses, becoming active in the church. The very first convert was a woman who ran a business selling alcohol on the islands. She immediately poured it all into the ground, giving up her livelihood, and put up a small house to accommodate visiting ECM workers.

So the church was established on Jana. From the very start it was essential it was regarded as their church, so a 'committee' of islanders was very quickly found to select people for senior positions and get training under way. We also left a full time worker in place to serve as a lay reader. Very soon the church became the focal point of the community and we started to think of building a school. A site was chosen, the islanders started to bring stones for foundations, and Evangelical Ministries organised a work team from N Ireland to carry out the building work. The team put up a well built single classroom which got the school started, and we built a house to accommodate the lay reader and a teacher. The work team got on well, especially considering all the difficulties of travelling and working in the very hot conditions there. One thing which puzzled them was the apparent lack of people – there was little evidence of the population we had been told about. Then, when ground was cleared and a football match organised, around 600 people turned up.

Following the model of what was done on Jana, we then began work on other islands too, and soon not only were there active communities and growing churches, but much more inter-island activity. This process of missions, establishing churches, organising training and starting schools continues steadily. Sport has been a big factor in bringing people together. ECM organised football and netball leagues, with inter-island competitions. This was taken very seriously, and the cup finals were a really big event with people travelling from different islands, and intense rivalries. Presenting the prizes after the competition was the government minister for ethics. He was so impressed with the work of ECM on the islands that he donated a boat. By this time we had our own boat but it was heavy, and not very fast. The new boat was fibreglass, much lighter, and is more effective for moving personnel around while the original ECM boat is based on the islands and can move big loads.

One very positive development we have seen on the islands and elsewhere is the developing relationship with government. We want to be able to hand things over to Ugandans rather than trying to keep on running them ourselves – with churches for example, they will be adopted by the Church of Uganda. The first school we built was on Jana – a single room. Very soon, the government built more classrooms and provided funding, while the school was administered by the Church of Uganda. This pattern was to continue with other developments.

Inevitably with all the health problems there, there are disabled children on the islands but it would be a long road to having the work of Cherub recognised and accepted there.

31.

BUKASA

Since the ECM work first started on Jana I've been able to make a number of trips to the islands. It can be an exhausting journey with a very early start, lots of preparations, lots to do out there in a short time, then the return trip. Patrick usually likes to pack into one day what others do in a week so going anywhere with him will always take longer than expected because, in addition to the main purpose of any journey, he will be taking the opportunity to do lots of other things too. So when Patrick gives the time for something, it doesn't do to take it too seriously!

At first, we travelled to the islands in hired boats. This was difficult; the boat wouldn't turn up on time, it might be smaller than expected, it could be slow and crowded, and we had concerns about safety. We bought life jackets to be used by our ECM workers in an attempt to minimise the risks. There were frequent accidents on the lake, with heavy loss of life. It was a big step forward when a donation enabled us to have our own boat built. This put us in control, we could ensure it wasn't overloaded and it was available when needed rather than having to wait at the lake for the boat we'd hired to turn up.

Even getting to the lake for the trip to the islands was difficult. The boats went out from Kisenyi, the main landing site for fishermen near Entebbe, but it was some way from the main road, approached by a very rough track. When we got our own boat Patrick was able to arrange for it to be kept at a lakeside resort, right beside the main road. This was a big improvement.

On my most recent trip to the islands in November 2004, we went in the fibreglass boat donated by the government minister. This made the journey much quicker. I travelled with Tommy Kerr and Fred Hand of Evangelical Ministries, who wanted to look at possibilities for future work teams. Also with us were Patrick, Sam, Denise, and Sam's daughter Ruth, as well as other ECM workers. Whenever Patrick goes, there will never be any empty space in a vehicle or boat. We were to visit a number of islands and stay overnight on Bukasa.

The day starts early for a journey like this. Although the boat is kept at the lake, the outboard motor stays at Patrick's. There were people to round up, load up the outboard motor, lifejackets, food etc. There would be supplies Patrick was bringing out to the workers on the islands. Then, so that films could be shown, we would need to bring a generator and other equipment. Finally, we'd go to a filling station to fill up the jerry cans with petrol for the boat.

When we got to the lake, the sky had clouded over and didn't look promising. The boat was brought in to shore, the outboard motor fitted, and everything loaded up. At last we got under way, and then the rain started. The first island we were going to was Jana. By the time we got there everyone was thoroughly soaked. There doesn't seem to be any method yet devised of keeping dry on those boats. It didn't seem to dampen anyone's spirits though. For the workers travelling out, this was a big day out, a chance to get away from the routine, to meet with colleagues. And in true Ugandan fashion any special occasion involved food, with different dishes being passed around the boat. For us, there was a sense of anticipation too, we were keen to see what had happened on the islands since we were last there and we hoped to be able to encourage the workers there.

We landed first at Jana and it was clear how happy people were to see Patrick. He's a remarkable character, able to go into difficult situations and take control. He has real authority and people respond to his leadership. It's hard to imagine anyone else who could have led the work on the islands or motivated people as he has. We walked to the centre of the island. When I'd been there before, it was just open ground. Now there was a school – the building put up by the work team, which doubled as a church, plus the classrooms built by government. We also saw the house we had built to accommodate the lay reader and teacher, who showed us round the school.

We then had lunch, joined by several of the first converts on the island who are now active in the church. By now the sun was shining, so we were able to take the money out of our pockets and leave it in the sunlight to dry. Everything was soaked, including the change of clothes I'd brought out in a small case.

From Jana we visited several more islands where we had placed ECM workers and another where we're not yet established, but there is great demand from the islanders to have ECM come there. They have seen what has happened on the other islands. Finally, after a long and tiring day we reached Bukasa island and started to unload the boat. We were met by Byakatonda, a former Besaniya boy who is now a teacher there. We were also met by Edmund, the ECM worker now serving as lay reader on Bukasa having recently moved there with his family. He and his wife formerly worked on Bubeke island providing strong leadership as the church was established there. I am always impressed by how the ECM associates are willing to go to work in these locations, it's very demanding.

There was accommodation on Bukasa. It's a big island, and a guest house had been built near where the boat landed. It was though at the top of a very steep hill, so we weren't finished yet. There is transport on the island too, one very old Land Rover. All the luggage and equipment was loaded onto the Land Rover, which left very little room for people, so most of us had to walk. It was now late in the day and all we wanted to do was rest, but it wasn't to be. We were no sooner into the guest house than Patrick called us all out and said we had to visit a school. We assumed he meant the local school, beside where we were staying, but we were wrong. We all climbed onto the Land Rover – thirteen of us. It was getting dark by now and we found that as well as having no roof and no brakes, the Land Rover didn't have any lights either. And so we set off across the island to the secondary school. It was a bumpy journey – when there's only one vehicle on the island, there isn't much spent on road maintenance.

We reached the secondary school to find the pupils had been waiting for us since midday – I think that wherever Patrick goes, that's the time he tells people he will be there! We met with the students, saw round the school, listened to the students singing, and Tommy Kerr was delegated to speak to them. We then thought, at last we can go and rest. But no, with Patrick we should have known better. He wanted us to go to Kisaba, the fishing settlement at the far end of the island, where they had run missions and the first converts were trying to get the church established.

We all climbed on to the Land Rover again and carried on through a forest in complete darkness. Presumably the driver knew where the trees were! The next problem was that we were driving across a plateau, whereas Kisaba was on the lakeshore. It was approached by a very steep hill – but the Land Rover had no brakes so couldn't go down the hill. It had to wait for us at the edge of the plateau while we all walked to Kisaba. Not only were we very tired, but because we hadn't expected to be out in the dark not one of us had a torch, and there was very little sign of the moon either. We had to stick close together.

I had seen a lot of places in Uganda but I'd never experienced anything like Kisaba. Around 1000 people living in dreadful conditions in a very small area. We could see very little as we tried to find our way through it in the darkness, but sometimes we'd pass a little hovel with a lamp lit and see six or seven people crowded inside. The place was also filthy. People must simply become numb to such conditions, and lose the will to do anything about it. It's not just poverty, as presumably the men were making money from fishing – but they spend it on sex and alcohol, leaving their families to endure these conditions. The social structures were breaking down too, and we were told that incest is common.

We eventually reached the 'church' where the converts had been waiting for us from midday. They had managed to put up four wooden walls (just a fence really) but couldn't afford to do any more. We were all standing in complete darkness but someone then brought a lamp from their house so at least we could see who we were talking to. It was late, so soon we started to walk back through the settlement. By now word had got round that there were visitors and a lot of curious people had come out – in the darkness we could sense rather than see them. Thankfully someone guided us with a lamp. A sick child was brought out for Denise to see – a little boy with spina bifida, reduced sensation in his legs, and because of this the rats had been eating his feet. This is something Denise could have dealt with in Cherub, the big problem is persuading the parents to bring the child or hand him over to us. I understand in this case that the child was eventually brought for treatment.

We made it back to the Land Rover and started the journey back across the island – a lengthy one, with several breakdowns. We just wanted to get to bed, but were taken instead to the school nearest the guest house where we were told a meal had been prepared for us. While we waited for the food (which arrived in a wheelbarrow) Patrick was setting up the equipment for a film show – but we had no intention of staying up for that. After the meal there were speeches relating to the school, church and community and finally we were able to get to bed. But it was going to take time to absorb all we'd seen that day.

Next morning we went to see the house we're building to accommodate Edmund. We also saw where an attempt had been made to put up a church building, but it had never been completed. We then went back to the boat and set off for Bubeke island where we were to attend church. This was under ECM leadership. After the service we met with a number of people, and a disabled child was brought for Denise to look at – severely deformed foot and ankle, and burns contractures. This boy was crippled, and yet could be treated in Cherub; it looked like his condition could be significantly improved. The parents obviously cared enough to want to do something for him but it has so far proved impossible to have them bring him to Cherub. This is why we need workers on the islands to build a relationship of trust and have people better understand what we are doing.

After visiting another island (Patrick is always moving equipment around and had to leave something there) we set off back to Entebbe. This time the sun was shining, and we had three hours of singing on the boat led by another Patrick, the lay reader who was returning with us to attend the ECM English classes. He also provided the musical accompaniment with a jerry can. They often sing choruses on the boat to lift their spirits. You start to worry though if they switch to hymns – that means there has been a change in the weather and they are starting to get worried! Conditions can get very rough on the lake.

We eventually got back, and we had a lot to think about. It was hard to take in what we'd seen on Bukasa, in particular at Kisaba. We'd seen the change brought about on other islands, but Kisaba was worse – what could we do there? We had Edmund on the island, but he was at the other end. He would visit to meet with the converts, but more was needed. We did however have generous donors who were usually willing to respond when a need was put to them – and we were aware of no greater need than what we had just seen.

What were we going to ask for though? Firstly, I didn't think anything could be achieved there till we had a full time worker. This would take time to arrange, so we got a donation to buy a motorcycle for Edmund. This let him visit more often to give what encouragement he could. We also needed to build a house for a worker. We wouldn't usually help with the cost of a church building, feeling that this is something people should do for themselves even if it's only four poles and a grass roof. Kisaba was a very unusual case though, and what seemed to be needed was a multi purpose building which could serve as a church, community centre, and possibly a nursery school.

So we knew what we wanted to do, but the donors we could think of were already helping us build houses and schools on several other islands so more help was needed if we were to deal with the problem effectively. Some time before that, Trevor Stevenson of Fields of Life had visited Nakapinyi and seen the needs of the refugees there. His organisation went on to build classrooms there. When he was there, Denise showed him the need for a community centre. When Denise, or Mary Mutumba, went there to work with the community they had to meet in the open air. Trevor went back to Ireland, saying he would try to find a donor.

Many months later Trevor got in touch to say he had a donor willing to pay for a community centre for Nakapinyi. I was delighted, and rang Sam Mutumba to tell him. Sam however was less than thrilled. He wondered if it was still needed. Since we had identified the need, Fields of Life had built classrooms and we were repairing the church building, either of which could serve other purposes. Our aim in any of the work is only to do what is necessary then move on to helping someone else. We hated the idea of turning down a donation, but didn't feel we could accept money to put up a building which could no longer be regarded as essential. I discussed this with Trevor. I knew he was already concerned about the islands, and I explained what we'd seen at Kisaba. He agreed to discuss this with the donor to see if they would consider helping put up a building there.

Thankfully, Trevor informed us soon after that the donor would help with a multi purpose building on Kisaba. Fields of Life would deal with all of this – they would go out and put up the building. This let us concentrate on finding workers and building a house. Things moved quickly (they usually do under Patrick's leadership). Working on the islands was new to Fields of Life, and they encountered a lot of difficulty – but they persevered. Patrick soon found a lay reader to serve there. A house was built for the lay reader, with additional accommodation for visitors. Next, two local people were employed as nursery school teachers and enrolment started. One year after identifying the need, the work is well under way and the Bishop of Namirembe consecrated the new church. At the other end of the island, where Edmund serves, his house is completed and the government minister who gave us the boat paid for completion of a church building.

We have seen that even in the most difficult circumstances change can take place. It's our hope and prayer that soon there will be a real sense of community there, enabling people to deal with their social problems. We've seen it happen on other islands.

32.

NAKAPINYI

It's beyond the scope of this book to consider in any depth what is happening in the north of Uganda, but it has been a deep frustration for us that we haven't been able to do anything to help there; it's astonishing to think that suffering on such a scale can be perpetrated over a long period of time without effective action being taken.   It's a massive humanitarian disaster which surely warrants international intervention, but it hasn't happened. The LRA has abducted very large numbers of children, brutalised and desensitised them, traded them as slaves, and forced vast numbers of people to be crowded into 'camps' for their own safety. Where this happens is a long way from Besaniya and we have tried at times to form links with people trying to work in the north but so far nothing has come of it. However the outworking of Cherub, going into the community to run clinics, brings various needs to our notice.

Nakapinyi, not far from Besaniya, is an area with sugar plantations which attract workers and came to our notice through Cherub running clinics there. The community is rather scattered, and we weren't at first aware of the diversity there. As well as the 'local' community, there remains the remnant of refugee groups who came there to escape the massacres in Rwanda. We then found there were also many refugees who had fled the LRA in the north. They were living in very crowded conditions, whole families squeezed into rooms built to accommodate plantation workers – and the influx of labour was keeping wages very low, resulting in many problems.

Having seen the problems, we wanted to help in some way. There were health needs which we tried to deal with through clinics, also issues relating to poverty which we tried to help with in a very limited way by distributing cooking pots, blankets etc. Of greater concern was the large number of children who weren't receiving an education. There was the usual problem of parents unable to afford to send a child to school. Even with supposedly free universal primary education, there were still charges to be met – very small by our standards, still impossible for many there. It wouldn't have cost us much to meet the cost of sending quite a few of them to primary school, but we would then have the problem of making them dependent on us. If we pay to send someone to primary school, very soon there is the expectation that we'll support them right through to university. We want to try to avoid getting into any more 'open ended' commitments, we have enough to cope with already. And there was another problem. If a woman with young children wanted to work in the plantations she usually expected the older children to look after the babies. This could be dealt with by arranging 'child minders', but there was still the problem of how to get the children to school.

Sam and Mary went regularly to Nakapinyi to investigate the problems. There were several schools there, so there seemed to be the capacity to get more children into education – but we didn't want to sponsor individuals. With one school, Sam quickly found the answer. Because of the long school day the children had to be fed – but the parents had to pay the cost. This would often be the child's only decent meal. Sam arranged to supply bags of maize direct to the school, and this immediately enabled the school to take in more children. He also helped in other ways - uniforms, books etc. This was the first step, but he then looked at another larger school. They had taken in a lot more children, but the school was desperately crowded and Sam estimated there were over 500 pupils and staff – and no toilets, with serious health implications. Once again, Sam decided the best way to help was by providing direct help to the school, so arranged to dig latrines. In doing this, he found another problem. The men in the area seemed to have very little motivation to do anything, and Sam had an uphill struggle to involve them – but he did, by among other things bringing bags of beans, and arranging football matches.

The latrines were built; it didn't cost much, and another problem was solved without us getting into any ongoing expenses. The government went on to provide further latrines, but the problem of crowding remained. Then Fields of Life, an Irish based organisation with a lot of projects in Uganda, came along and built more classrooms. There was another 'spin off' for our work when Trevor Stevenson of Fields of Life visited, and we discussed the need for a building to serve as a community centre. Trevor found a donor but by then we were repairing the old semi-derelict church, and that plus the new classrooms meant there was no longer much need for a separate building as a community centre – but the donor agreed to build instead a multi-purpose building at Kisaba, which is described elsewhere.

There were people from different areas living at Nakapinyi, speaking three different languages. Some had spent their whole life there, others were recent arrivals. There seemed to be some degree of mutual tolerance, understanding and respect, but the rapid growth meant fragmentation, some were becoming isolated, and there needed to be some focus to again make it a community.

Again, the Mutumbas came to the rescue. The clinic visits helped in gaining an understanding of the problems; the home visits and follow ups in particular let us see the problems people faced there. There was an established church there, meeting in a classroom as the church building was almost a ruin, but everything there was stretched to the limit, and the lay reader alone couldn't deal with it all. Mary Mutumba then started going regularly to meet with the women. I had the opportunity to see her women's fellowship there – she had managed to bring them all together despite their different origins and languages, and they were thoroughly enjoying engaging in a range of activities. This seemed to set them on the road to becoming a 'community' again, which made a big difference to the quality of life there.

Some time later I attended a Sunday service there, conducted by the visiting archdeacon, and I met a number of the local people including community leaders. The church service (in a very crowded school classroom, with many people outside) was well attended by all sections of the community, and there were a number of speeches afterwards. These made clear just how much the refugees had been welcomed into the community. In such a poor area, there could so easily have been resentment. What happened there was an education for us in how direct personal involvement, and help with some simple and basic projects, could make a big difference. It cost very little, and soon our work was done and we were able to move on. We retain a limited link now with occasional visits, but can seek to apply the lessons learnt to other projects.

One problem which was evident at Nakapinyi, and which we don't know the answer to yet, was how to involve the men. When Mary organised the women's fellowship, the women were really eager to attend. Sam however faced real difficulty in trying to motivate the men. As a result we have been looking since then at how we can develop a men's ministry, and at getting the men to face up to their role in family, church and community. We also see big problems with the men on the islands and are presently deciding what we can do, the first step being to come to a fuller understanding of the problem. With ECM a lot of the work in local churches etc involves women; we also have a separate child evangelism team visiting schools. The next step is to have a men's ministry. Like many other agencies a great deal of our work is with women and children – they certainly encounter a lot of problems which we want to address, but the men are all too often the cause of the problems so in a way we have been treating symptoms rather than providing a cure.

33.

THE CURSE

Life can be hard in Uganda. A family with a disabled child can face an uphill struggle, it's tough when someone isn't able to fend for themselves as most people struggle to deal with their own needs without having to care for someone else. Of course there is the extended family which can take care of orphans, but even that system is breaking down with the spread of Aids. Orphans though can still do their share of the work, whereas the disabled may simply become a burden. For this reason, a family may see no other way than to starve a seriously disabled baby to death. There's a lack of knowledge too, and we don't need to look too far back to see similar attitudes in our own society. The disability may be seen as a curse, perhaps it's a result of something they have done in the past. It can be a stigma on the whole family. These are some of the attitudes which need to be addressed, and while the problem is widespread I wouldn't want to give the impression that no one cares for a disabled child. As well as many difficult cases, we also encounter parents who against all odds are doing their utmost for a disabled child. In some of the cases we have seen the conditions they have endured have left us wondering how the child has survived up to now.

As Cherub became more widely known, so it was more likely that children would be brought to us. Particularly in the early days, and still in some areas, it was a case of following up on rumours of a disabled or injured child. Sometimes too a lack of knowledge led to suspicions about our motives; a lot of sensitivity was needed to persuade someone to hand over a child to us and while the treatment in Cherub was usually very successful, we had to be careful about people's expectations and remember that things could go wrong too. Thankfully very little has gone wrong, and the successfully treated children have encouraged others to come.

The very first club foot patient admitted to Cherub was a neighbour of Sam Mutumba in Luweero, a boy of around 10 years old. Sam referred him to Cherub when he started looking around on behalf of Cherub – till then, he hadn't known that his neighbour had a child with two club feet as he would have been kept in the house. He was successfully treated and can now lead a full and normal life.

We are based at Mukono, a large town on the main road about 11 miles outside Kampala. There are missions and government health services in the town and surrounding area, but even there we find cases, just a short distance away, of people, for whatever reason, not being brought for treatment. One such was a boy of about 12 whose bowel was exposed and discharging openly from birth. Because of this he was kept at home; we don't know why his family never sought help, they may have thought or may have been told that nothing could be done for him. There are many 'traditional' doctors people may turn to, whose advice may be very questionable. This child was referred for surgery, treated successfully, and can now go to school and do the same things the other children do.

We have had children come into Cherub who the parents had effectively rejected and we always had to be careful about the kind of environment a child was being returned to. We sometimes had a lot of work to do with the family, but usually realisation would dawn that despite the disability, this was a child like any other and it was wonderful to see an emotional bond forming that wasn't there before. We would see parents who simply didn't know what to do with a child begin to take a very close interest in their treatment in Cherub.

For many cases surgery wasn't appropriate. There is a lot of cerebral palsy and lack of knowledge leads to a continuing deterioration, with the child tightening up and movement becoming more and more restricted. But effective physiotherapy can help a great deal. We have seen children enabled, in a very short time, to stand upright and walk perhaps for the first time. This on its own won't be of much value unless there is continuing care when the child returns to the community, so the parents need to be trained and know what to expect. I have seen caring mothers absolutely delighted to find that there is something they can do for their child.

I don't want to give the impression that no one else was doing anything about disability in Uganda. Others had been working for years to deal with various problems before we came along, but what was done fell far short of the countries' needs, and large areas were well beyond the reach of the existing services. The Uganda Orthopaedic Project was an exciting development, able to have an impact on a national scale. As 'beginners' in the field it was essential for us to be part of a larger programme; we depended totally on their back up.

We hope and expect things to be different in future. Increased knowledge, better facilities, more widespread access to medical services mean that conditions such as club feet can increasingly be treated at birth. Other problems relating to malnourishment, infection, improperly administered injections etc should diminish. But there is a big backlog of cases to deal with and Cherub should be very busy for years to come.

It's a big boost for Cherub when a child completes their treatment and returns home. Often the change in them is dramatic, and everyone can clearly see the difference. Sometimes a child can be in Cherub for a very long time. One such child, suffering from osteomyelitis, was responding to treatment but still had a long way to go. Because he had already been away from home for so long, the decision was taken to take him back for a visit so that everyone could see the progress. He had a leg in plaster, but was able to walk with crutches. The villagers' reaction was unexpected – they were horrified and frightened. It seems when they saw the plaster they thought we had replaced his leg with a white one in an attempt to change his colour. This was a timely warning that we still had a lot to learn, and had to take more care about how we were perceived.

34.
AIDS

It's hard to write anything about the work in Uganda without touching on the subject of Aids. The work of Cherub isn't directly linked in any way with Aids but other parts of our work are, and it's like a shadow over everything that is done there. Often unseen, but inevitably having an impact on just about everything from the economy through medical work to education and the church.

There is almost a sense of unreality about it. Walk through Kampala, see the signs all around of an active, crowded vibrant city with a growing economy, then consider the percentage of the people you see who will die of Aids, who are already HIV positive. They look healthy, and may remain fit for some time, but then comes the rapid deterioration, the part most visitors don't see. It's bad in the city, but so much worse on the islands. How can we prevent children following the same path? The causes are well documented, but prevention difficult. Of course there is widespread education, and safe practice is encouraged – but we are dealing with human nature, compounded by a 'live for today' attitude, not helped in many cases by a poor quality of life. Add alcohol to the mix, and it's clear education alone isn't the answer. Many of those contracting HIV are educated and know the risks they are taking. Most of the time they wouldn't dream of taking risks; but then there are the vulnerable times, when their guard slips.

As well as doing everything possible to educate, and prevent the spread – in our case mainly through literature work, or on the islands for example by improving the quality of life – we have to deal with the aftermath. People who know they are going to die, and who are unable to provide for their children. Aids doesn't kill one parent, it kills both. A steeply increasing number of orphans to be cared for by the extended family, and that structure itself breaking down as more and more are affected. So many families now cared for by the very young or the very old, with seriously inadequate resources. What means they do have often used up in an attempt to provide medical care for the dying. Family land sold to raise money for treatment – taking away their only means of support for the future. A bleak picture, yet largely unseen in places because of the veneer of activity and development.

In the Besaniya Children's Home, most of the children are Aids orphans, some abandoned by parents who knew they were dying. We also have links with child headed families, where all the children are also HIV positive. There is little we, or other outside agencies, can do when faced with a problem on this scale, their own extended families and communities must support them, but there are limited ways in which we can give help and encouragement.

It's hard to look at the present situation and see what the future holds. Someone who is now HIV positive, with improving symptomatic treatment, could live for 5 years, 10 years or more before becoming ill, so the present situation doesn't give a true picture of the eventual impact. Uganda is far from the worst affected country, having introduced an Aids programme at a relatively early stage, but vast numbers will still die, leaving a massive orphan problem. And behind these numbers, every individual case is a human tragedy.

Thankfully we have moved on to some extent from the awful problems caused in the past by a lack of knowledge; people afraid to do anything to help Aids sufferers, people wrapped in sacks and left outside to die, the judgmental attitude of those who felt it was their own fault and therefore didn't feel obliged to help. We still see the dreadful situation of men seeking to remain safe by having sex with younger and younger girls in the hope they won't be infected. We have also seen very effective work done by locally organised voluntary groups working in the community, the encouragement given to a household with an Aids sufferer when neighbours offer to help instead of shunning them.

But whatever the positive and encouraging signs, there is a massive problem, increasingly sapping the resources of the medical services and aid agencies. The statistics are unreliable, the percentages affected vary enormously between urban and rural areas, trade routes or places like the islands. Accurate figures are difficult to ascertain, even the experts find it hard to agree. Of course education and other measures taken to limit the spread are having an impact, but it is still a big problem. I spoke to staff at Aids clinics, and they said they are still not seeing a decline in the number of people testing HIV positive. It's tragic to see so many young people in particular with a death sentence hanging over them, and so many parents having to suffer as they care for their sick children who had sometimes gone on to successful careers but then came back to the village ill, and watch them die one by one, often their whole family wiped out, leaving them to care for grandchildren in their old age.

Drive or walk through Kampala and you will see little of this, it's a country of such contrasts. Then take the time to look beyond the superficial, to see the problems encountered, and try to think what you can do to help.

Through our work with the church there, it's our hope that we can tackle causes rather than just symptoms, and see the people themselves changed. Instead of preaching safe sex or trying in other ways to avoid becoming infected, they will be fundamentally changed and adopt Christian standards and values.

Consider the following words written by Catherine, who found she was ill when she had a medical examination prior to leaving for the UK to complete her doctorate:

"The world had stopped moving for me. I couldn't accustom myself to the thought that I was not travelling to Britain...... A month later, other signs of Aids had shown. I was too depressed to live alone and returned to my parent's home. I could not eat or sleep. I could not pray. I was lost in a maze of dark thoughts.

"I thought about life. We spend so much time planning for the future. We become so preoccupied with our plans that we never give God a glance. Somehow we struggle through and maybe once in a while go to church on Sunday and that's it. We put God aside and leave him there, yet He says He created us so that we live our lives for him. 'For thou hast created all things, and for thy pleasure they are and were created' (Rev 4:11). In my loneliness and despair my thoughts about life would seize me and hold me captive for hours. As the various symptoms of Aids took their toll on my progressively wasted body, I thought more and more about life.

"I began to realise that I had turned away from what God initially planned for me. I had also ignored the good work that Jesus Christ did for me on the cross. I was running around chasing the desires of my heart, every day of my life, forgetting about God.

"Aids is a disease which demonstrates that our physical bodies are secondary to our souls. 'seek first the Kingdom of God and the rest will be added unto us' (Matthew 6:33). Many of us have ignored this and concentrate our efforts on trivial earthly matters. Before I was thirty years old I was a lecturer at Makarere University. This was a source of pride for me and my family. I had concentrated many years of effort to achieve this. But I used none of this success to glorify God. With Aids, there was nothing to show for it. Remember that this body you work so hard to please will one day rebel against you. Our parents are grieved with the loss of one child after another. They have been so busy making their children's lives comfortable they have ignored the God who gave them this gift.

"We are all guilty of ignoring our creator. The devil rejoices in this situation and lays snares for us. I pondered on these thoughts, but I told no one. I was so scared of death, so scared of people's reaction to the fact that I had Aids........... I knew that Jesus was the missing link in my life. When I asked God to forgive my sins because I accepted that Jesus died for me, there was always another voice saying, 'No shame? After all you have done, now you go back to Him? It takes a lot of washing to clean you.' I had a lot of problems believing that the blood of Jesus could really wash me clean without me earning it. The next thing I wanted so badly was to do some work for Jesus. My works could never earn me salvation, but they became a response to all Christ had done for me.

"Having gone through this depression and overcome it only through giving my life to Jesus Christ, I had decided to use the remaining period of my stay here assisting those who were facing this period. I lived every day with the hope that I would one day help people overcome the depression that follows acquiring Aids by telling them about Christ and what He came to do.

"I plunged into giving this testimony to all my visitors. It was exciting to be useful again, after all hope had been lost. Many visitors came to see me during this period. But eventually I exhausted my circle of friends and family. I still wanted to work for the Lord and reach many other people who could not come and visit me. I decided to write.

"It's sad that it takes something as devastating as Aids to help us face the purpose of life, but living to please ourselves is already the worst sort of death. The only way we can have life, both here and through eternity, is to come into a right relationship with God.

"Along with Paul I say that:

Philippians 1:20-23

20. My deep desire and hope is that I shall never fail in my duty, but that at all times, and especially just now, I shall be full of courage, so that with my whole being I shall bring honour to Christ, whether I live or die.

21. For what is life? To me it is Christ. Death, then, will bring more.

22. But if by continuing to live I can do more worthwhile work, then I am not sure which I should choose.

23. I am pulled in two directions. I want very much to leave this life and be with Christ, which is a far better thing."

35.

CO-OPERATION

In November 2000, when Norgrove Penny showed us round the recovery ward at Mengo and we saw the children who had undergone surgery the previous day, I remember seeing one little boy who made a big impression.

Often it could be very tedious work preparing materials to send out to Uganda. It took a lot to fill a container, and often there would be months of work bringing in equipment, scrapping a lot of it, and preparing what we thought was worth sending. Loading a container was hard work too. We were paying for the volume so wanted to pack in as much as we possibly could. Sometimes it was boxes of books or medical consumables – that was easy, we just kept stacking them in and mixing the box sizes to fill the space. Other times it was much more tricky – large pieces of medical equipment which might be very heavy or fragile. We had to secure them, then work out what to pack round them to fill the space. It became a big three dimensional jigsaw puzzle. What kept us going was the hope that everything sent would be of some value, and occasionally we heard about how it had been used.

The medical equipment was hardest to deal with, particularly when we had large quantities of orthopaedic equipment which was often only of use as part of a 'set'. We spent many hours going through medical catalogues trying to work out what we had, what else needed to go with it, and whether anyone could actually use it. We also knew the cost of some of these items, so felt it was worth taking the time to try to find a use for it. A lot of the equipment we had sent out over the years had gone to Mengo, and I would see much of it in use as I walked round the hospital. We had helped supply a number of departments. Norgrove was able to show me how some of the orthopaedic instruments and supplies had been used, and told me of one particular item.

The little boy we saw in the recovery room was probably about seven years old. He suffered from TB spine, which meant several of the vertebrae had collapsed, trapping the spinal cord so that he became paralysed. In the early stages this could be operated on. In this boys case the fear was that it had been left too late. The other problem with spinal surgery was that an implant was needed – a Harrington rod – and these were much too expensive to be used in Uganda. I had absolutely no idea what a Harrington rod was, but it seems that while we were usually thorough in checking everything we sent to Uganda, a box of these rods had been included in one of the consignments without us realising – either that or I thought they were for something else! Because of this, a Uganda surgeon operated on the boy's spine. As he lay there, it was too soon to tell what the outcome would be but I later heard that the operation was successful and he was walking again.

I have great admiration for the skills of a surgeon. I am often fascinated to see what surgeons, or other people with particular skills, are capable of doing, but which I couldn't possibly do myself. Yet here was an example where, in addition to the skill of the surgeon, a whole chain of people was involved and it reinforced the value of those long hours spent sorting and packing. It was a useful reminder that in mission work there is a role for everyone. We shouldn't simply think "there's nothing I can do."

I've no idea now where that box of implants came from, we often get surplus equipment from hospitals. But someone in a hospital had called us to offer equipment, others had helped me to go to collect it. Then someone helped sort and pack it all. We then had to find people fit enough to load it all into a container. Someone provided the cost of shipping the consignment to Uganda, and when it got there others, on our behalf, had to unload it all and direct it to its intended destination. Some of our workers there also spent many hours dealing with all the customs formalities. Finally those implants reached Mengo, and thankfully someone recognised them instead of them simply being put to one side and forgotten about. Still more people were involved, as a skilled theatre team backed up the surgeon in completing the operation. It's a clear example of how we can collectively achieve something which wouldn't have been possible for us as individuals.

This is the kind of image we try to keep in mind as we deal with the more mundane day to day work. We've since heard of other cases where lives have been saved or transformed through a piece of equipment we have sent out – it might have been something apparently very modest, of no great value, but was in the right place at the right time. I hope such stories are an encouragement to all who help us but don't have the opportunity to see the results.

36.
WHO PAYS?

We believe all our work in Uganda has been exceptionally cost effective; real change taking place at minimal cost, and particularly low administrative costs. In fact most of our administrative costs are covered through direct gifts or other means, so we can usually guarantee that any money given to us can be used in total for the designated purpose.

It takes time to build an effective support base. My first experiences raising money for work in Uganda related to short term projects – help with water pumps for Mengo Hospital and, later, sending a container. We also occasionally raised money for small projects such as publishing a book. This was relatively easy; we made needs known through our own church, friends and acquaintances and, having dealt with the projects, there was no ongoing commitment. But things soon changed. Our initial personal commitment was to Mengo and having become involved, we didn't want to suddenly stop. We went on to send containers, also air freight consignments of drugs or equipment, and helped with their water supply. We were fortunate that some of those who helped with the initial projects were willing to continue helping, and understood the needs.

It was a big step becoming involved with Besaniya – although at first we had only intended helping with administration, not becoming fund raisers. At the start, Africare's understanding was that we would help with child sponsorship if another donor could be found to pay for the buildings. This didn't happen and we ended up raising money for all the Besaniya work. This was a time of great need in Uganda, and we started to find people willing to help. It wasn't always easy though. I was doing a full time job as well as raising money for Besaniya. I was also still trying to provide ongoing help for Mengo Hospital and starting to help with the setting up of ECM. These were 'personal' projects which at that time were entirely separate from Africare, and it was demanding keeping up with it all. I should say though that after what we had seen in Uganda, we were committed to doing whatever we could. We soon found that it was much easier to raise money to pay for something – a building, piece of equipment, or vehicle for example – than to fund an ongoing work with no apparent end to it. Some people are cautious about getting into long term commitments. Others like to help with something more 'tangible' than ongoing costs. Despite all the difficulties the work grew, and more people joined us. It wasn't easy. We had determined workers in Uganda wanting to get on with things and we wanted to encourage them, but Besaniya in particular was very 'stop-start.' Often building had to stop because money wasn't coming in quickly enough. But, as the first buildings were completed, children moved in and people could see it all taking shape, the support increased.

Of course the aim with Besaniya wasn't to put up buildings, it was to help children, and we only had a small number in the home. We then started to help more children through an external sponsorship scheme and as money came in we started to help more and more children. This stretched us at times. School fees rose, and we also had to contend with people's expectations; if we helped with primary education they wanted us to continue through secondary and beyond. There were children we agreed to help for a short time, but they quickly forgot it was a limited agreement. This caused problems, particularly when funds were short and we had to apply strict criteria. We wanted to help the most needy, but a lot of people thought we should be helping them when we didn't feel their cases were a priority.

Despite these difficulties, the scheme in general worked well and a lot of children were helped – but administration in Uganda could be very hard work if we were to ensure that the help went where it was really needed. Some people were much better off than they wanted us to believe. On other occasions we found 'phantom' children appearing on the list, or schools trying to charge us higher than normal fees. We depended very much on our Ugandan workers checking everything carefully.

We were grateful to the increasing number of donors willing to give regularly, covering Besaniya running costs or paying children's school fees.

Unless in exceptional circumstances we tried to avoid linking donors direct to an individual child. We didn't want a child to know they had a sponsor, as they could become much more demanding and effectively we could make them beggars when they should have been doing more for themselves.

Our approach now is changing, and particularly since we started work with Cherub we have been cutting back on external sponsorship and finding other ways of helping – like building schools or helping with community projects that can help larger numbers. Now that so many more Ugandan children have access to education, it was right for our work to move on, and we are thrilled with what Cherub is now achieving for children who might otherwise have been almost without hope. We do however try to remain flexible and continue to help some children with vocational training, if they face some difficulty, or if the skill they are training in seems worthwhile. We also have our scholarship fund, set up in memory of Fred Masumbuko, to help selected students through university.

The cost of the work has grown too and from small beginnings we are now spending much larger sums of money. There have been big donations along the way which have made some of the significant 'steps' possible, but also a large number of smaller donations. Each donor individually may not give much, but collectively it has made it all possible and we have needed every one of them. It is this large number of regular donors who enable us to meet all the running costs.

So where does it all come from? Often the larger sums have been donated by personal friends; some were friends when we started, others we met through the work and became friends. It meant a lot that people had sufficient confidence in us to donate these sums. We also occasionally received help from donor agencies, some for a project, others providing regular support. Some money has come in as a result of taking meetings in churches or with other organisations. The bulk of it though comes in response to either circulars or personal letters. We have always felt it important to keep people fully informed of what we were doing with their money.

As the work grew over the years, we often had to do things we found difficult. For some things we hadn't the necessary experience, but still had to do it. At other times we found ourselves in situations we could never have imagined. Yet despite all our inadequacies the work grew. It brought with it a range of new responsibilities, mainly to those working for us in Uganda. The biggest responsibility though was being entrusted with other people's money. It would have been so much easier to spend our own money; spending other people's money meant we had to do everything possible to ensure it was used correctly, in the way they intended and to maximum effect. There also had to be total transparency and Hazel spent countless hours dealing with the detail of the accounts. We are especially grateful for always having had professional accountancy help on a voluntary basis – this has ensured we can satisfy all accountability requirements, and also avoid fees.

Nothing stays the same. For years, the income kept increasing as the work grew. To some extent the work is as big as we can satisfactorily manage, but we were also aware that there had to be some limit to our income, and it eventually levelled out. In part this is because we are running out of people to ask, but the main reason is a significant change that has taken place in the way churches and others support overseas work.

It's a shrinking world. Advances in communications and transport have opened up previously unimagined opportunities for direct links with other parts of the world. This can be a very positive thing enabling us for example to react more quickly and effectively to need. It can be negative too, when people react too quickly without an adequate understanding of a situation, or perhaps for the wrong motives. It is too easy for us to make people beggars when we don't take the time to understand traditions or culture, or think we know best how to resolve a problem. When we started helping Mengo there were very few others doing anything similar and we had no problem getting large quantities of equipment or supplies to send out. For years most of the hospitals' surplus came our way. With Besaniya, there were few other similar projects supported from here, and quite a few churches and individuals worked with us. Same with ECM, this was something new which caught people's imaginations.

Soon though more and more people started travelling as previously inaccessible countries opened up. They formed personal associations in these countries, they brought information back to their own friends and churches, and soon there was a dramatic increase in the number of projects supported. This has of course had a big impact on the support we can hope to receive, but I am not complaining as it's wonderful to see so much taking place, and to know that we helped many other people get started. Through sending out work teams or passing on equipment to other agencies, a much broader work developed. There is a lot we aren't directly involved with now, but there are examples where we were in 'on the ground floor' and it is pleasing to have seen some good ideas become reality. The whole background to our own work is difficult though. There have been big changes here, with available resources (whether it's money or skills) being shared around an unprecedented number of projects. Uganda has changed enormously too, and our work must reflect these changes.

It is still our hope that as long as we ensure we are reaching the neediest with our work in Uganda there will be those people who will identify with us and help us make it possible. We constantly review what we are doing, and are increasingly using the experience of our workers in Uganda as the basis for making decisions about the future. We are in a situation now where we usually try to end one commitment before engaging in another one; we want others to take responsibility instead of always depending on us. Where we do want to see growth continue is the work of Cherub. There is no one at present to take over our responsibilities there and we want as much help as possible not just to continue the work but to keep standards high. We want to effectively treat disability, but we also want Cherub to continue to set standards and be an example to others.